How Can You
Help Me
If You Don't Believe
Me?

Biography of a shaken patient

Dianna Wood

Order this book online at www.trafford.com
or email orders@trafford.com

Most Trafford titles are also available at major online book retailers.

Printed in the United States of America.

ISBN: 978-1-4669-4668-2 (sc)
ISBN: 978-1-4669-4667-5 (hc)
ISBN: 978-1-4669-4669-9 (e)

Library of Congress Control Number: 2012912617

Trafford rev. 12/06/2012

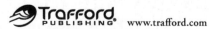 www.trafford.com

North America & international
toll-free: 1 888 232 4444 (USA & Canada)
phone: 250 383 6864 ♦ fax: 812 355 4082

Contents

Introduction vii

Chapter 1   My Family History 1

Chapter 2   Childhood.. 11

Chapter 3   My Teen Years 23

Chapter 4   My Twenties 38

Chapter 5   The Thirtieth to Thirty-fifth Year 55

Chapter 6   The Diagnosis, Denial, and Acceptance 68

Chapter 7   And the Diagnosis Is Definitely,
            Well Maybe, Could Be 73

Chapter 8   Cascading Effects from Loss of Dopamine.............. 90

Chapter 9   Meanwhile, In My Ordinary Life............................ 98

Chapter 10 The Ethical Relationship between the
            Patient and Insurance Provider........................ 106

Chapter 11 The Ethical Right of a Patient to a Diagnosis........ 129

Chapter 12 The Ethics of Advocacy or Can a Patient
            Be His Own Advocate? 153

Chapter 13 The Self Advocacy Groups Still Don't
            Get the Message 170

Chapter 14 Whose Life Is It Anyway?................................ 185

Introduction

I have lived with Young onset Parkinson's disease for twenty years. This chronic disorder has forced me to make my health a full-time job. I read all the current research and technological resources available to make intelligent and ethical decisions regarding the health care treatment I receive. Because I am the only person who is experiencing my symptoms, I frequently have "clashes" with my health care team regarding both the diagnosis and treatment of my illness. I want to give up the fight and just let the health care system determine my care but must remain ever vigilant not to fall into the cracks.

Parkinson's disease, according to the *Merriam-Webster's Medical Dictionary*, is "a chronic progressive disease chiefly of later life that is linked to decreased dopamine production in the substantia nigra and is marked by tremor and weakness of resting muscles and by a shuffling gait." Is "Parkinson's disease" a disease or just a similar group of symptoms shared by many different persons of all ages, primarily aged, who for several different reasons lose the functioning of their dopamine-producing neurons?

Dopamine is an inhibitor of serotonin, a pleasure neuron, causing the patient to suffer from anxiety and depression. Also, dopamine and serotonin are both neurons that regulate the appetite center of the brain. In addition, the reproduction hormone prolactin, regulated by the neuron dopamine to encourage milk production in women, is overproduced. Dopamine also fills the eye lens and stabilizes the shape of the eye. Lack of dopamine can cause premature retinal damage. This makes the possibility of making a correct neuropsychological diagnosis extremely difficult. The diagnosing physician must rely on the patient's personal health history and clinical observation for a diagnosis.

The question the diagnosing physician must answer is if the patient has one disease with cascading effects or specific damage to the nervous system caused by damage to the spinal cord or/and brain. Is Parkinsonism not a disease but just a group of symptoms created from different causes?

If the patient does not prepare him/herself with a list or notes of all his/her symptoms and relies strictly on the neurologist's power of observation derived from his/her years of experience, chances are the diagnosis may end up incorrect. The most current research states that after studying the brains of persons who died with a Parkinson's disease diagnosis, 15 percent were misdiagnosed. No two neurologists have exactly the same patients with the same symptoms.

The experience of diagnosing Parkinson's disease can be different from one physician to the next based on the different symptoms or stage the patient is in. How can all different neurologists come to the same diagnosis after seeing the same patient without the differing experiences? Why is there a higher incidence of the disease in the Northern States rather than the Southern states?

Symptoms appear after the initial disease has already destroyed 80 percent of the dopamine-producing neurons. Is it possible the initial cause is as unique to the patient as the disease is itself?

Parkinson's disease is currently diagnosed based on the patient having two of the three major symptoms: Tremor, rigidity, and bradykinesia. "Other diseases which are also diagnosed as Parkinson's disease are Essential Tremor, Multiple System Atrophy, Progressive Supranuclear Palsy, Dopamine responsive Dystonia, delayed stress syndrome and Restless Leg Syndrome." One woman was diagnosed with "Conversion Disorder" ("a psychoneurosis in which bodily symptoms; a paralysis of the limb(s), appear without physical basis.")[1] Now isn't that an easy out for the overworked doctors? The doctor cannot detect the patients' problem in the initial ten minutes spent with the patient and he knows he must diagnose the patient or order tests. If, as neurologist claim, there is no test for Parkinson's disease, how can they claim the patient has "Conversion Disorder?" Are the doctors calling their patients liars? It brings to my mind the image of the movie *Sixth Sense* when the child patient asks Bruce Willis, who plays a child psychologist, "How can you help me if you don't believe me?"

The diagnosing physician has only the patient's history, the patient's symptoms, and today's technology as evidence to confirm his diagnosis. When one neurologist may diagnose the patient as having "Conversion Disorder" (based on only his opinion from the neurologist's past experience) while a different neurologist may believe the patient's symptoms are real and diagnose the patient with Parkinson's disease, which neurologist is the patient to believe? The doctor may insist the illness is in the patient's head or a conversion disorder. The problem is that "Conversion Disorder" and "Depression" and "Anxiety" may be treated one way and Parkinson's disease is treated another. The doctor may treat the poor woman as having Conversion Disorder, discover his diagnosis was incorrect when the symptoms do not lessen but increase, and diagnose the woman with a different neuropsychological disorder. The patient, diagnosed with Parkinson's disease by a different neurologist, could not know which neurologist had the correct diagnosis. Also, the psychological damage could cause depression and anxiety. After which the neurologist will attribute the depression and anxiety felt by the patient as part of the Parkinson's disease.

Treating the neuropsychological symptoms is like the little Dutch boy putting his finger in the dike when it sprang a leak. More and more water began to flow out of other areas of the dike until the water pressure overwhelmed the dike. Treating the patients' symptoms as they appear will help their quality of life at first. However, when drugs are prescribed for the patient's symptoms it is just a matter of time until the body rebels and puts the patient's life in jeopardy.

Knowing the etiology of the illness and being able to point to which gene has a mutation and at what point in the genome chain or what toxin the patient was exposed to will enable researchers to name the patient's disease and begin research for a cure based on scientific facts, not guesswork. There is much comfort knowing the symptoms you are experiencing are not just "in your head." Relying solely on a neurologist's clinical diagnosis leaves you open to having that opinion overthrown by a second neurologist's diagnosis at any time.

Many neurologists see no reason to have better diagnostic tools and place all priority for research funds to finding a cure. I am a patient who benefited from current technology to prove I had Parkinson's disease by an F-DOPA PET scan and by a commercially available genetic test. I am a great promoter of genetic research. Gene research is a slow and cumbersome process as every small step to discover the protein the gene produces also uncovers a chemical process as to how the protein affects other proteins produced by other genes. The research is slow and requires careful documentation, but may lead to a cure because all steps are scientifically proven.

There is only one commercial DNA test available for persons with Parkinson's disease provided by Athena Diagnostics which enables the patient who has the test to know the results. Most patients, because they cannot afford to pay or their insurance will not pay for the test, end up joining a research group to have their DNA tested and are never aware of the results. To be a member of a DNA study requires the patient to sign away all rights to any information obt from a DNA test obtained for research. This practice denies the patient information that might help to make decisions about what treatment is best for their individual type of disease.

Many of the current treatments for Parkinson's disease were stumbled over by accident, including the newest surgery to install Deep Brain Stimulators. In addition, many of the funds for research used to find a cure are guesswork. There is no "norm" for Parkinson's disease. Adding to the confusion, many different movement disorders fall under the name of idiopathic (of unknown origin) Parkinsonism.

Up to this time, etiological research (to determine specific attributes of the disease) has been done at Universities and Hospitals around the country. The pharmaceutical industry was not allowed to spend money on television advertising and spent next to nothing trying to raise funds to do etiological research. Money was made treating symptoms, not curing the illness itself, placing the pharmaceutical focus on the symptoms not the cure. Most medical research money came in the form of government grants awarded to colleges and other medical educational facilities. Patients with illnesses also banded together and raised funds to pay for research.

When Christopher Reeve tragically fell during a jumping competition and broke his spine, suddenly the whole picture of research was changed. America is a consumer society, and Reeve used his fame as an actor, and his power as a consumer, putting all his talents into becoming a "self advocate" for those with spinal injuries. With the use of his money and his ability to understand and find the most current research, he nobly tried to aid victims of spinal cord injuries by beginning a not-for-profit patient advocate organization.

Christopher Reeve, with the best intentions in his heart, began to accumulate a huge sum of money. His organization educated patients on spinal cord disease and provided grants, which changed the research industry, rocking health care providers to the core and changing the tide of ethics and politics in research. In his eagerness to find a cure for his illness via stem cell research, he insisted that grants be written to encourage stem cell research because it had the *potential* to help all sorts of neurological disorders. Understand, please, that I am not calling Mr. Reeve a liar, but question his scientific basis for including Parkinson's disease as one on those possible illnesses.

Pharmaceutical companies began courting his organization as well as the many other new advocacy groups springing up. Michael J. Fox started a nonprofit organization to beat Parkinson's, as did Muhammad Ali. Several consumers with neurological diseases began to start small organizations called patient advocacy groups or grassroots organizations to advocate for the particular disease they were afflicted with and lobbied to persuade state senators and representatives how to vote for health care bills. Pharmaceutical Companies support the American Parkinson's Association and the National Parkinson's Foundation as well as many of the smaller Patient Advocacy Groups by providing free educational brochures and sponsor educational workshops at which brochures about their products that would help Parkinson symptoms are prominently displayed.

The concept of each of these advocacy groups is to educate and support patients as well as raise funds for research. Most were funded by Pharmaceutical Industries pouring more profits into advertising on television and providing tax-free literature to nonprofit educational workshops and less money into research.

More and more responsibility fell to the FDA for research grants to pay for research. Funds were diverted to rising neurological illnesses caused by veterans exposed to the horrors of war, new chemicals made to spray on produce to kill weeds and insects, and seepage of chemicals into the water supply.

A new industry of "nonprofit" organizations of patients politically lobbying for consumer-defined health care was born. The pharmaceutical companies worked hard to convince the nonprofit advocacy groups to award grant money to their companies, thereby letting consumers be in charge of what the pharmaceutical companies would study.

Pharmaceutical companies advertise their products by offering free T-shirts with their company logos, pens, pencils, coffee cups, and coupons as a way of free advertising at educational get-togethers or fund-raisers by patient advocacy groups. I personally have received an extra long Shoe Horn, a digital clock, and numerous pens, writing pads, pillboxes, and T-shirts from pharmaceutical companies. Much of the grant requests specifically appeal to the emotional side of advocacy board members. The majority of patients, with firsthand experience living with the disorder, were used to raise money, but given no say in how the research money could be spent.

According to CNN, "The branch of stem cell research was well funded by the Christopher Reeve Foundation. Spinal Injuries are extremely complex injuries. It is a condition that affects one American every 49 minutes. The Christopher Reeve Foundation (CRF) occupies a unique position in the spinal cord research community. Since 1982, it has aggressively pushed all accepted boundaries by seeking out the best and brightest scientists and encouraging them to tackle the enormous challenges of spinal cord repair. CRF's research philosophy is bold, forward-looking, and strategic."[3] Mr. Reeve claimed stem cells were his hope for a cure. He spoke out in an interview on CNN with Amos King. The words in italics are my own comments.

> KING: You mention 100 million Americans. *[The American census of 2006 counted 245 million Americans, including children, so is Mr. Reeve stating almost half the population has a spinal injury?]* This is a debate in which just in this program we've heard the voice of the pope, voice of many of the politicians in Congress.
>
> It's also a debate, though, with many personal stories, including yours, and from the world of Hollywood and celebrities. Michael J. Fox has testified before Congress saying he believes this research could help cure a disease he has, Parkinson's disease. *[What was Mr. Fox's medical evidence for this conclusion? Was he merely influenced by Mr. Reeve's belief in the miraculous claims of stem cell potential?]* Jenny Tyler Moore has gone before the Congress and said perhaps in stem-cell

research, including embryonic stem-cell research, is the cure for diabetes. *[Medical research does back this claim up as growing a new pancreas or liver is not as difficult as programming stem cells to build neuron pathways specifically for dopamine to pass through.]*

Tell us in your case, sir, how do you believe that this research could specifically perhaps help you?

REEVE: Well, in my case, I suffer from something called demyelination. Moreover, that means that, in one very small segment of my spinal cord, about the width of your pinky, the coating, myelin, which is like the rubber coating around a wire, has come off. And that keeps signals from the brain from getting down into the body.

So the human embryonic stem cells could be cultured and then sent right to the site, and they would know that their job is to remyelinate. And then the signals from the brain would go down properly, and I would get recovery of function.

But let me say that I think this research is important not just for people with spinal cord injuries, but let's just take the case of people that have ALS, Lou Gehrig's disease. There's no cure for it whatsoever. And it is always fatal within two to six years. The body just generatively falls apart.

Now, what a couple of researchers did recently is proof of principle, which is very, very important. It was Dr. Gerhard and Dr. Kerr at Johns Hopkins, and they were able to inject mice or rats with a virus which simulates ALS. They then injected human embryonic stem cells. Then, over a period of time, the progression of deterioration was stopped, and all the rats showed recovery of function.

Now, that is proof, because some people say, well, we don't know what embryonic stem cells can do; it's never been proven. Well, that's a huge first step. And of course we won't know what they can do until we go and do the work. But the work must not be stopped, absolutely.[4]

According to the Christopher Reeve Foundation website,

Patient advocates of several neurological diseases, admirers of Christopher Reeve, took up his banner to crusade for funding for stem cell research for all neurological illness without medical evidence that the stem cell treatment option was the best option to follow. They also did not advocate for a better life quality for those living with Parkinsonism in the here and now. There was little advocating for more research for genetics that could be the best research to discover the etiology of how neurological systems work. The patient advocates, who were not medically trained, could not explain the scientific aspects of how stem cell therapy worked. The self advocates instead emphasized the morality of stem cell research. The advocates were very successful when they changed the focus from if research on stem cells were scientifically feasible to if it were morally ethical by man's standards. They argued the embryos of abortions were just being tossed as trash. Why should this valuable resource be discarded when it could save lives?

Stem cell lines may provide replacement parts for simple organs. Scientists are limited in their ability to direct a stem cell to differentiate into specific tissue of cell or cell types. According to J. Eric Smith, PhD, MD, director of the Movement Disorder in Mayo Clinic located in Rochester, Minnesota, "The brain is not simple. Trying to program stem cells for specific tasks is analogous to replacing microchips in a computer (not just a diode or wires, but complex interconnected circuits.) Fetal transplantation experience suggests that stem cell transplantation will be a disappointment."

He goes on to report of two controlled clinical trials with the same results from (federally funded) Fetal Transplantation for PD.

"Fetal midbrain containing dopamine neurons transplanted into brains of people with:

1. Parkinson's Disease (fetuses 6-8 weeks gestational age)

2. Some received "sham" surgery as control group

3. Fetal dopaminergic neurons re-populated the patients' striatum.

4. Benefits were modest at best."

Dr. Smith's conclusion was that "stem cells have no capacity to restore complex brain circuits."[5]

The Parkinson patient advocacy groups continue to press for stem cell research by moral arguments. They press the pharmaceutical organizations to continue research of embryonic stem cells as a possible cure. The Pharmaceutical companies see the dollars being thrust at them to pursue this line of research and could hardly be expected to say no to the consumer. They have continued researching embryonic stem cells with no positive results for the millions spent, which they continue to receive from not-for-profit advocacy groups. I attended a workshop designed to persuade Parkinson's patients to advocate for embryonic stem cell research as well as to keep the current federal funding to the Veteran's program because, as the blond who was in charge of the workshop stated with a wink, "That's where the money is." I was appalled at her brassy attitude and her assumption that everyone in the room must agree with her. Many religious people do not. Two faiths are firmly against the use of embryonic research: the Catholic and Evangelical Lutheran faiths.

Due to the emphasis on stem cell research, other potentially beneficial treatments are not being pursued. For example, a group of patients recently received stem cell growth factor (GDNF) to increase the number of dopamine-producing cells in their brain. I believe them when they reported immediate improvement. The study was suddenly discontinued with no reason given to the recipients of the growth factor. Patients, who went from being bedridden to walking while taking GDNF, went back to being bedridden when it was withdrawn. The self-advocate group, PAN, immediately insisted that the pharmaceutical company resume the delivery of the growth factor via a shunt that had been surgically placed in the subjects' brains for delivery of the growth factor. They lost the case.

Many of the self-advocate Parkinson's disease patients blamed the pharmaceutical companies for not continuing the research for financial reasons. Many self advocates encouraged patients to stop participation in research studies. The result of such a stubborn and shortsighted outlook would shoot themselves in their own feet by slowing the search for a cure. The goal was to see if GDNF worked (it did), but the delivery system caused harm to the patients. Patient advocates chose to overlook the contract signed by each candidate of the drug trial that they should not expect to benefit from the study. Their participation in the study was to benefit those who followed them. Much as I empathize with the patients involved, it wasn't their time to be the first to benefit from the research. Still many patient advocates wish to force the pharmaceutical company to provide the drug for patients because of the pain and suffering they underwent by having the brain surgery to insert the shunts. Perhaps research contracts should be reworked less in favor of the research groups and more in favor of the patient.

For my part, I support adult stem cell research as I know a dear friend who had a daughter diagnosed with a deadly form of leukemia after only one year of marriage. Without the research done on bone marrow adult stem-cell therapy, the young woman would have lost her life. Adult stem cells were placed by an IV drip into her system after she underwent several radiation sessions to kill her own white blood cells. This beautiful young talented woman is now living a productive life, and her young husband is relatively sure he will be able to grow old with his bride.

Since the etiology of Parkinson's is still unknown, there is no way of determining the long-term effect of the delivery of embryonic stem cells into a Parkinson's patient's system. Researchers of the Parkin 2 gene have found patients with mutation(s) are focusing not on the dopamine-producing neurons as the factor in Parkinson's disease but on the delivery of the dopamine to the muscles. "Our experiments demonstrate that the directed expression of the parkin gene counteracts the PD-like symptoms in the *a-synuclein*-induced *Drosophila* model of PD. Manipulation of the ubiquitin/proteasome degradation pathway in such a specific manner apparently remedies the toxic accumulation of *a*-synuclein. This study demonstrates the success of selective targeting of toxic proteins for degradation as an approach to address neurodegenerative conditions such as Parkinson's disease. The development of therapies that regulate *parkin* expression or parkin protein activity may be crucial in the treatment of PD."[6]

Essentially, the study states that the dopamine-producing neurons, even if replaced by embryonic stem cells, would only continue to die because the dopamine was destroying itself. The dopamine produced by the neurons was backing up on itself in the substantia nigra part of the brain. The tangles of protein (produced by the mutation) were clogging the delivery pipes.

Health Maintenance Organizations (HMOs) have sprung up across the country in an effort to hold down medical costs for the consumer. Consumers run these organizations. The doctors no longer cannot obey the Hippocratic Oath and the guidelines of HMOs on what prescriptions can be prescribed or tests may be given. Specialists, such as neurologists, base their diagnosis on the experience they have had over the years. But the different illnesses in the brain of many patients have unknown causes. What one neurologist has experienced as delayed stress syndrome can be identified by a different neurologist as Parkinson's disease. Patients must begin to educate themselves about their symptoms and understand what their symptoms mean. Patients, not the doctors, should manage their own health care to receive the most benefit from treatments for neuropsychological diseases because of the complexity and unknown etiology of the working of the brain. Patients may not advocate as a group in the health care system because each patient is unique in the symptoms they experience. Patients must stop blaming the pharmaceutical companies and the medical community and take responsibility for their behavior as self advocates and for the lack of knowledge regarding the etiology or knowledge of how to treat advanced Parkinson's sufferers. The pharmaceutical companies have spent billions on stem cell research at the request of the self-advocacy groups. No benefit or benefit for very few are now turning blame on the pharmaceutical companies. Self-advocacy groups are calling the pharmaceutical companies greedy for attempting to fill the self-advocacy consumer market demands.

I have lived with this ethically flexible and challenging system for twenty years. Because of my full-time commitment to understand the most current information and my refusal to allow any professional to tell me the symptoms I experience are untrue or false, I have maintained my sanity with a dash of humor and continue to exercise my right to influence research by my government-given right as a consumer.

Being a patient advocate means taking on responsibility, as well as power, to change pharmaceutical research. I would prefer to see research focus on the cause of Parkinsonism more than chasing possible scientific-based theories. I have learned to live life to the fullest with the disease and have dismissed thoughts of dying of the disease. I encourage other patients living with any neurological illness to empower themselves by educating themselves about every aspect of their illness. This is the only way they can be sure that their diagnosis and treatment are correct. No two people diagnosed under the Parkinson's disease umbrella are exactly the same.

Neurologists do not have the needed information to treat their patients as of yet. The workings of the brain affect the entire body, and the neurologist must be educated about the cascading effects of the neurons and proteins and how they affect the rest of the body. Much of this knowledge has not been uncovered at this time. Knowing where in the brain the damage begins is not enough to treat the whole patient.

Patients should also begin to take a serious look at the current research protocols. As things stand now, all the benefit goes to the research team and none to the patient. I would particularly challenge the NINDS right to withhold the information disclosed to patients who offer a vial of blood to test DNA.

I chose to ask for my genetic testing done by a corporate entity, not as part of a research project, and I know the results of my Parkin2 genetic test. I was able to use the results to prove I had Parkin mutations. In the summer of 2005, I was placed in a coma on two separate occasions to clean my blood of the toxins built up by the use of Sinemet, the current gold standard of treatment for Parkinsonism. These toxins were destroying my kidneys. I did research on the internet of studies done for persons who had my mutation and proved to my neurologist that DBS surgery was my best option to lower my intake of drugs. The research studies I found stated that I was a particularly good candidate for this procedure. I had the procedure done despite the negative response of my neurologist. The movement disorder specialist based her reasoning on her experience with patients who had undergone the procedure. She was afraid that my history of depression and anxiety could cause me to commit suicide. I assured her that I was a strong Christian and could not consider suicide because it was a sin. I explained to my doctor that she could not base her decision on her past experience with other patients because I was a unique individual. I am grateful that she allowed me to take the risk of having the surgery. It saved my life. I have cut my meds to about a third of what I took prior to surgery. None of this would have been possible if I hadn't kept up to date on the research and sought all available technology, especially DNA test results, to confirm my diagnosis.

There should be a check box on every DNA research form allowing the patient the choice of knowing or not knowing the results of the test. This information belongs to the person who donated their blueprint of who they are and the information should be theirs to use as they wish outside of the study. It affects the patient's ability to make health decisions in life. Is there a possibility the gene would be passed on to his/her children? They have the right to use the information of their DNA to choose to have or not have children. Whose life is it anyway? The researchers should also include a paragraph of what their plans are for the information they collect. If the purpose is to copyright it and earn money off of whatever genetic line they have studied, the patient should know. If their purpose is to share their knowledge they compiled with other researchers, patients should know. Have any gene lines been copyrighted that could answer questions being studied by other research groups? If the information obtained from DNA research is copyrighted, rather than shared, the cure for many diseases will not be available until the copyright is no longer valid. Medical costs will escalate for the patients who need genetic-based treatment. Medical researchers are in a new era of discovery. Only if patients refuse to cooperate with research groups who are out to profit themselves at the expense of many ill Americans will ethics overcome the corporate allegiance to the almighty dollar.

Notes for the Introduction

1. *Merriam-Webster's Medical Dictionary* (Merriam-Webster Inc., 1995), 138.
2. 2005 Government Statistics, Table?
3. King, L. CNN interview of Christopher Reeve.
4. King, L. CNN interview of Christopher Reeve.
5. Smith, E. PHD, MD, Presentation at 2004 Parkinson's Update, in Minneapolis, MN. Copied from Printed Handout.
6. Haywood, A. and Staveley, B. BMC Neuroscience Volume 5, 4/16/2004, *Parkin counteracts symptoms ina Drosophila model of Parkinson's disease* *http://www.biomedcentral.com/1471.2202/5/14*

Chapter 1

My Family History

My very first childhood memory was of being in the living room of the house I grew up in. I was alone, in the dark living room, when suddenly there was a sharp flash of lightning followed by a loud crash of thunder. The lights went out, and I ran terrified and screaming to find my mother and two older sisters in the TV room. I spent the remainder of my childhood in fear. I mention this because stress is considered to be a cause or possible major effect on Parkinson's disease.

My mother was born Marie Sue Lyndale Tenyson to a Lou Tenyson Lyndale Black. Her father is unknown. Lou was married to Thomas Lyndale and had two children older than my mother: Thomas Lyndale Jr. and Lindsey Belle Lyndale. J. T. Lyndale, Thomas's father was a horticulturalist for the University of Michigan in Ann Arbor. Lou Tenyson was descended from a long line of Irish Great Lake Sea Captains and was born on Harson's Island in St. Clair, Michigan. Lou's father was Ernest Tenyson, killed prematurely when struck by a city bus on his own street.

FATHER OF 5 IS KILLED WHEN BUS STRIKES HIM.

Ernest Tenyson, 46 years old, of Halsey [now known as Royal Oak], Michigan, the father of 5 children died today in the Highland Park General Hospital of injuries suffered yesterday when he was struck by a motor bus at Main Street and Council Avenue in Halsey. The driver, Carl Gibbon, of Birmingham, was not held.[1]

His widow, Jenny Stella Hogan, was Lou's mother. Lou was their eldest child. Shortly after Ernest died, Jenny Estelle (Stella) gave birth to the last of Ernest's children, a daughter she named Stella. The daughter was born on July 31, 1926, and died at five months of pneumonia.[2] Prior to that, on May 17, 1926, Stella Tenyson, thirty-six years old, was declared to be feebleminded by the Pontiac State Hospital "based on a psychometric tests, has a MA of 9 years, and an IQ of 59+."[3] All her children were removed from her home. Lou, being the eldest, was already married to Thomas Lyndale.

The second eldest was Leonora Tenyson, aged 16, who was placed as a maidservant in Halsey and was married a few years later to an aviator who was killed in World War II."[4]

Next was Frederick William, ten years old, who was placed in a state school for a while until a relative took him in to work on their farm. He was later killed in action.

First War Dead Arrives Friday

Military Services for Pfc. James W. Tenyson to be held Monday. The remains of Pfc. James W. Tenyson, brother lived with Mrs. Justice Black of Algonac, (Lou) who met his death in the Normandy invasion, July 27th, 1944 are scheduled to arrive in Algonac tomorrow, Friday, Dec. 19th from the Distribution Center in Columbus, Ohio . . . He is survived by his mother Stella Tenyson of Cement City and three sisters. Mrs. Black, Mrs. Lee Stokely, Mt. Clemens and Teresa Tenyson of Coldwater. Funeral rites to be conducted by Rev. G.M. Houghton will be under the auspices of the VFW Post 3901 and American Legion of Algonac and will be held at 2:00 p.m. Monday at the Gilbert Funeral Home with burial at Oaklawn Cemetery.[5]

The next child was Teresa who was also declared feebleminded and placed in a state school in Coldwater Michigan.[6] As an adult, she retained employment at a motel in Algonac, where she remained most of her adult life until the motel burned down. She was then placed in subsidized housing. She died in a nursing home in East

China Township, but I was able to visit with her once a few years before she died. She was quite confused and thought she would be released to her apartment the next day. She talked a little about my mother's mother and some other family members. My mother was not interested in getting to know her biological aunt.

> Teresa G. Tenyson died Sunday, September 26, 2004, in Medilodge of St. Clair.

> She was born June 3, 1921, in Algonac. She is survived by her sister, Terry Borgert, brother, Frank Swihart, and her niece, Sharon Leeth. Funeral services will be 1 PM Thursday in Algonac Church of Christ. Minister Thomas McNerney will officiate. Burial will be in Oaklawn Cemetery, Algonac. Visiting hours are 2 to 4 and 6 to 9 p.m. Wednesday in Gilbert Funeral Home and noon to 1 p.m. in the church. Memorial donations may be made to the Algonac Church of Christ. The last children were Frank Tenyson and his sister Terry who were both adopted by the same family.[8]

If you count the children accounted for by the Pontiac Mental Hospital, you will notice that although the news article stating "Father of 5" didn't match up with the seven children accounted for. I can only assume Stella had two children who were not the legitimate offspring of Ernest Tenyson. I also learned at a later date that Stella Tenyson had sixteen surviving children.

I was able to find both my mother's half siblings from her mother's first marriage. Thomas Lyndale had married a Gina Lyndale. He already had a daughter named Tanya Lyndale who committed suicide in her thirties by an overdose of heroin. She had been diagnosed with multiple sclerosis before her death.[9] Thomas was also deceased. Lindsey Belle is alive and well, living in Alaska. She had not known she had a younger sister when I contacted her while she was eighty-two. Both she and my mother are deaf and correspond by mail. They have yet to meet in person. Lindsey Belle sent pictures of herself to me, and we look like we could be twins.

My biological grandfather, Ernest Tenyson, was a sailor. His father, Bruce Tenyson, was a Great Lakes Ship Captain. He married Bertha Platt. "They lived in the family home on Harson's Island. The island at the time had no more than fifty residents, and the roads were unimproved dirt ones. It did have a park, Tassmoo Park, which attracted three excursions that shipped regularly to Harson's Island, making the city of Algonac known as a summer resort town.

Bruce Tenyson had a small motorboat to bring the family to town to shop, but he always anchored the motorboat quite a distance from town and made the family walk to Algonac to do their shopping. It seemed that he had a good deal of trouble starting the little motor on the boat, and being a lake captain, he had a certain litany of words he went through every time the motor failed to start. He didn't moor the boat in town because there would have been too large an audience for him to start his motor in his usual fashion.

"Captain Bruce was a pilot who was quite superstitious. When he was eighty-seven he was called on to act as honorary captain of a ship which had lost its captain in Detroit when he was taken sick and had to go to the hospital. He took the ship through to Duluth, MN, where it was headed, but refused to go back with it on its return voyage. He said he had a bad feeling about the boat. He was right. It broke in half and capsized on the return voyage."[10]

My mother never knew anything about her biological family and only cooperated with my research because I felt it was important I know my family's health history. She was adopted by Zeke Edison, an engineer for the Detroit Edison Power Company. He also owned a building built to be two flats. My mother, renamed Jenny Lou, and her father lived upstairs, and the bottom level was rented out. Her father was married three times before settling on his former ex-neighbor's wife, Micky. Micky already had two children: Terry and Butch. My mother felt like Cinderella. She felt her stepmother didn't love or fairly treat her as she did her own children. My mother was especially at odds with Terry. Both my mother and her stepsister fell in love with the same man named Tom. According to my mother, Terry, who was older than Tom, falsely trapped him into marrying her by telling him the lie that she was pregnant with his child.

My disappointed mother began spending more and more time working on her most current love, riding horses. She spent a lot of time in Saginaw at a horse riding ranch called Wagon Wheel, and it was there that she met my father. After a whirlwind courtship, they were married on New Year's Eve in 1948. My mother has a picture of her in her tiny dress on her petite five-foot frame with my six-foot-tall strong and trim father in his army uniform, with hazel eyes and wavy black hair as they were cutting their wedding cake.

Before my father was shipped to North Korea, my mother was pregnant and living with her new mother-in-law. She tended bar at night to raise money for herself to try to meet expenses. When my oldest sister was born, my mother told me she was disappointed because the baby slept most of the time and never stayed awake long enough to play.

"My father was struck by a missile in North Korea on June 4, 1951 and was sent home to recover for a while before returning to duty."[11] My father had not been present for the birth, and when he first held my oldest sister, she cried being unfamiliar with a male voice. My mother told me the war changed my father. He was sadistic and would humiliate my mother. My mother was confided in by my father's foster sister that he had been sexually abusing her from the age of five. She offered no help or belief. Before he returned for active duty in Korea, he managed to impregnate my mother again, and my second sister was born in August of 1952. She was an independent, assertive, and strong-willed person—everything my mother wasn't. My mother was very proud to have a daughter so much stronger than herself. My father was still overseas at her birth, and once more, both girls cried when he came home, being unused to the male voice. As my middle sister grew, she tried to please my father and earn his praise by being the best at everything. Unfortunately, it only made my father try harder to make it impossible to please him.

My father, if he were changed by the war as my mother said, ended up being a dominating, sadistic man. His father, Joseph Jerome Fischer was born of Irish descent.

One of the places where my father's ancestors lived was Albert Lea, Minnesota, where my great grandfather John grew up, met and married Grace Carpenter, who died an early death at childbirth. His second marriage was to a Janice Pugh. They chose to leave Minnesota and continue toward the west. In Castlewood, South Dakota, Janice gave birth to a son, Joseph Jerome Fischer, my grandfather. The Fischer family continued to migrate to the west and finally settled in Clallam County, Washington.

Logger Dies of Injuries

Joseph Jerome Fischer, 27, of Sapho, succumbed at a local hospital at 1:55 o'clock this morning from injuries received Monday when he was hit by a cable in the Sapho camp of the Bloedel-Donovan Logging Company. Fischer was a rigging slinger and had been employed by the Bloedel-Donovan Company for the past five years.

Born at Castlewood, South Dakota, October 26, 1906, the late Mr. Fischer came to Bellingham when he was 6 months old and moved with his parents to Maple Falls shortly afterwards and lived there until entering the employ of the logging company there. He was married to Sarah Kenney at Maple Falls, May

22, 1926. The widow and three children, Carolyn Jane 6, John Joseph 4 (my father); Peter Jerome 2 survive. Other survivors are his mother, Mrs. Janice Nelson, Maple Falls; two brothers Justin and James of Granite Falls and three sisters; Mrs. Jack Spratt, Bellingham; Mrs. Dennis Frost and Rachelle Nelson, Maple Falls.

Funeral Services are to be held in the chapel of the Dewey Lyden Funeral Home here Saturday morning at ten o clock. Burial will be in the Maple Falls cemetery at one o' clock Sunday afternoon.[13]

Sarah, now a widow with three children, was living with her mother-in-law when tragedy struck her life again. Her sister, Lelia Kenney, 20, died from a basal fracture of the skull received when she fell from a slow-moving automobile.

Sarah found the memories of the recent tragedies too much to bear and moved herself and her young children to Saginaw, Michigan, where she resided with relatives until she met and wed a farmer and set up house on a farm on Genaw Road. My father does not talk about his past much but obviously did not like his new stepfather. At some point, his stepfather died, and Sarah married an Ivan Morrow whom I knew as my Grandfather my whole life. My father constantly made fun of him, but he provided my Grandmother with a good home. My father adored his mother even though she rarely smiled. I remember little of her except she was a wonderful tailor. She used to make doll clothes for my dolls, and she also taught me how to color.

Because of the genetic component in my case of Parkinson's, I was curious whether any of my ancestor's had the disease. I wondered if my mother's niece, Tanya Jeanne Lyndale, who committed suicide at age 33 after being diagnosed with Multiple Sclerosis, might have actually suffered from early onset Parkinson's. Similarly, my sister Annette had been diagnosed with MS before receiving a diagnosis of Parkinson's Disease.

Notes

1. *Detroit News* dated January 7, 1926.
2. Pontiac State Hospital Letter dated May12, 1931.
3. Death Certificate, County Troy, MI dated January 24, 1927 Michigan Dept. of Health.
4. According to the *Detroit News* dated January 7, 1926.
5. Algonac, St. Clair County, Michigan, Thursday, December 18, 1947 paper.
6. Pontiac State Hospital Letter dated May12, 1931.
7. Algonac Courier, Tuesday, September 28, 2004.
8. Pontiac State Hospital Letter dated May12, 1931.
9. Death Certificate, State of Nevada, Vital Statistics Doc. # 003903.
10. Harper, N.G., *Interesting People* Interview of Lenore Chapman Tenyson dated Thursday, May 30, 1974, Pg. 6 Algonac Courier.
11. Government Online Records for Korean War. 5th Ca Regt (Inf) Div.
12. Port Angeles Evening News, 2 Nov, 1933, P.1 col. 7.
13. *The Everett Daily Herald*, Nov. 29, 1933.

Chapter 2

Childhood

After the war, my father, who is very quick in Math, went to work as an apprentice for a tool and die maker called Fischer Body Company in downtown Detroit. My mother was pregnant but was very unhappy to have another child. She felt trapped in a marriage that didn't give her any love, respect, or freedom. My father was a dictator, kept her in the dark regarding finances, and did his best to shame her into staying in the loveless marriage. He was very pleased when I was born because he was finally able to hold a baby who didn't cry at his voice.

The family my father now had had grown too big to continue living at his mother's farm and the farm was too far away from where he worked. My father found a big old house in the city of Roseville, Michigan, and that was where my family lived when I was born.

We lived there for about two years. Then my father bought a new rambler-style house in the suburb of Clinton township. The house had three bedrooms, a family room, kitchen, informal dining, formal dining, living room, a full bath, and a half bath. The lower level or basement was unfinished. It also had an attached two-car garage. To my mother's delight, she discovered an old school friend lived across the street just five houses down. We children were also able to walk to the elementary school about three blocks away. It was in our new house that I had my first memory of the lightning/thunder scare

When I was frightened by the bolt of lightning and crash of thunder, I must have been three or four. My father worked the afternoon shift, from 2:00 PM to 11:00 PM, so I rarely saw him. But on weekends, he made his presence known. It did not take much to inspire his wrath. He would hit our bare bottoms as punishment for what would normally be considered normal childhood play. If we played in the backyard on the grass, walked on the front yard grass, walked one step off the boundary of the sidewalk onto a neighbor's property, left our room to play with a sister in her room, or did not eat everything served for supper, we were soundly spanked. Both of my sisters hated green onions, so father would force them to eat extra helpings. When I reached school age, I could smell a block away when my mother cooked liver with onions and would begin crying the rest of the walk home. I usually threw up the liver, but my father would make me sit back down at the kitchen table and eat another piece until I kept it down.

On every Thanksgiving, a meal we were expected to eat until our sides felt ready to burst, there was some pumpkin pie left over one year. It was not placed in the refrigerator but sat on the counter a few days and developed green mold on it. Our father made each of us eat a piece of it, telling us it was good for us because the mold had penicillin in it. There were three very sick young girls that night.

We were not allowed to have friends in the house when our parents were not home, for that matter, it was a rare occasion any friends would come to the house if they knew my father was there because they were also afraid of him. My oldest sister had a friend named Sue, and my other sister had a friend named Michelle. One day, my two sisters had their friends in the house when my parents were out. For some reason unknown to me, they all began to fight, tearing the bedding off each other's beds and tearing clothes off the hangers in the closet and throwing games out onto the floor. While all this was going on, I snuck into the house, famished, and grabbed a couple of Ritz crackers to tide me over to dinner, knowing we were not allowed to snack between meals. My father was working the day shift by then. He came home while my sisters were still fighting. I felt a sick feeling in my stomach even though there was no way to be connected to the mayhem as I was sitting obediently on the front porch.

My father ordered my sisters' friends out of the house and ordered my sisters to clean up their rooms. He then came out and ordered me into my room. He then made all of us sit in our rooms for three hours without dinner anticipating the punishment that was to come. He then entered my eldest sister's room and proceeded to spank her bare bottom (she was fifteen by this time) forcing my middle sister and me to listen to her cries of pain, knowing our turn was coming. He then entered my other sister's room, and proceeded to do the same to her (she was twelve). By the time he entered my room, I was terrified. I hadn't even participated in the mayhem, but he spanked me regardless just in case I had been involved.

Another time, he had painted the coat closet door and I accidentally touched it, leaving my fingerprints in the paint. Terrified at what he would do, I lied and said I had not touched the paint. But as the paint was oil-based back then, I had been unable to wash the evidence completely off my hands. He soundly spanked me twice: once for touching the paint and a second time for lying about it. I never lied again.

During all our elementary school years, we were not allowed to associate with either sister; we were not allowed to watch more than one program a week. Rain, snow, or shine, we had to spend at least an hour outside, usually on the concrete porch, either sweltering in the sun or shivering in the snow.

The beginning of my first grade year found me in a special reading class with one other person who also could not read. By the end of my first grade year, I was top in the class and won the spelling bee. I loved my first grade teacher, Mrs. Foster. She inspired me to read by letting me sit on her lap as I sounded out words in my soft, unsure voice.

When in the house, we were not allowed out of our rooms, not even to talk to each other. I read constantly: Nancy Drew, Trixie Beldon, Annette Funicello, and eventually moved into biographies of scientists, explorers, presidents, and numerous other famous people.

Summer vacations were a month of misery. My father now received four weeks of vacation, and he was promoted to foreman. By the time I was eight years old, he was moved to the day shift. My mother would take us clothes shopping in the last two weeks of July. I was always a disappointment to my mother because I hated to shop. We would pack the new clothes into suitcases and just drive across several states. If we came to a state park, we would rush through it, snapping a few pictures, jump back in the car, and drive for another eight or nine hours before finding a cheap motel room for the night. I saw all forty-eight states of the United States (save Hawaii or Alaska) and remember nothing about any of them. I remember seeing mountains, some green with trees, others made up more of rocks and sand, but could not tell you which states the mountains I saw were in.

Sitting in a car for long eight-hour stretches of driving is not easy for three young girls in the backseat with no air-conditioning. My father was constantly reaching around to smack one of the cranky daughters across the back of the head, and things would be quiet for the rest of the trip that day. When he hit you, it would cause you to black out and see stars for a while.

One particularly grueling summer after having driven for a few days with no stopping for stretching or exercise, I became very constipated. After having our usual big breakfast at a Pancake House restaurant, we started off. A few hours later, my stomach was becoming extremely queasy. I was too frightened of my father to ask him to stop and threw up my breakfast in the backseat. He stopped the car by the side of the road, pulled me out, and spanked my bottom hard as my mother and sisters cleaned up the backseat of the car. When the backseat was as clean as it could be made, we were herded back into the car. I was given a bucket, and we continued on our way. I continued to vomit every hour or so for the rest of the day. When we finally arrived at a motel that night, I was miserable and exhausted. My father forced me in the bathroom, made me pull down my panties, and stuck his finger up my rectum to see how constipated I was. Then he went out and bought some Milk of Magnesia. He gave me two large spoonfuls of the chalky stuff and then I was left alone in the room while the rest of the family went to dinner. I began having severe stomach cramps about 9:00 PM and was up and down all night, either vomiting or having stool movements sometimes both together. By morning I was exhausted. When we went for breakfast, my father ordered me a bowl of prunes. Despite my mother's pleas to give me a day to recover, my father insisted that we had to keep moving to see all the sights he had set out for that summer. Since we only had pit stops when the car ran out of gas, I was forced to sit with stomach cramps, unable to relieve myself for hours, waiting for the car to run out of gas.

When I was nine years old, our house was struck by a tornado in July. I had just gone to bed at the time and heard what sounded like a freight train and felt the whole house shiver. I could hear my parents shouting at each other as they went around the house closing the windows. A few minutes later, my mother came into each of the children rooms and led all of us to our back door. When she opened it, we all were shocked to look up and see stars where the garage roof should have been.

The rest of July was spent walking around on the hot shingles of the collapsed garage roof, pulling out nails from the shingles and stacking the shingles in the backyard. We also had to use a hammer and chisel and knock the cement off of what remaining bricks were able to be reused. Of the two cars in the garage, our station wagon (fondly nicknamed the Bomb) was totaled, and the 1954 Buick, brought home that very day the tornado struck, having had a new paint job, was repairable.

My father took my mother on the back of his motorcycle and went to a Cadillac dealer to buy a new car to replace the totaled Station Wagon. None of the sales staff working the floor bothered to talk to the two leather-jacketed people who were checking out the cars on the showroom floor. Finally when my mother saw a powder blue caddie she fell in love with, a salesman walked over to check the leather-jacketed couple just to be sure they were not looking to steal a car. He would not let them test-drive a car unless he rode along. When they got back to the dealership after the test-drive, my father said he would pay cash for the car. The salesman laughed, thinking my father was joking but was suddenly silent and much more respectful when my father handed him the wad of bills necessary to buy the car.

Despite the damage to our home that summer, my parents continued with their plans for a vacation in August. All the necessary clothes shopping was done; the bags were once more packed, and we were off for a rare stay in one state, Florida, for two weeks. The last two days of the vacation, a hurricane made its way to Fort Lauderdale, where we were staying at Henry's Hotel. We had a room on the second floor facing away from the ocean, so my parent's chose to wait it out. The day the hurricane approached was windy, and the waves in the ocean were huge. We did not dare go into the ocean with the strong undertow caused by the increasingly higher waves. We were able to find more shells that last day than we had found during the rest of the two weeks we had spent there as the ocean waves continued to dump onto the shore the treasures from under the sea. Hurricane Cleo struck the shore at Fort Lauderdale that evening. Looking out the window, it was like a fireworks display with all the electrical wires whipping around in the wind. We lost our power almost immediately. Two single women with a room on the oceanside lower level made their way to our room and requested to stay until the end of the storm. Permission was granted and no one slept that night. Even though we were on the second floor facing away from the ocean, we still found ourselves stuffing towels under the door to keep out the water and sand being pushed in by the high winds. We were fortunate that none of our windows were hit by the coconuts that were being pulled off the palm trees and hitting the building like missiles. Eventually the wind quieted down, and we could see stars overhead. We found ourselves in the eye of the storm. This period of the storm lasted about ten minutes before the wind began whipping up again with its whistling and thunderous forceful noise. The storm was over by morning.

The hurricane left behind a great deal of sand, flooded roads, coconuts, and broken power lines. The sign with the name of the hotel had fallen on our brand-new Cadillac. We packed up our things and collected a bunch of the coconuts that had been blown off the trees. All three of us children had managed to develop ear infections from swimming in the ocean, so all the way home, my parents were forced to listen to our cries of pain. The cries grew particularly loud whenever my father would lower his window of our now air-conditioned car and throw out his burning cigarette butts. They were blown into the backseat. They would land and burn the occupant of the seat behind him, which granted him no end of perverse pleasure.

While still discussing my childhood years, I would like to mention my father's strict belief in the philosophy that children were to be seen and not heard. Anytime my parents were visited by family or friends, we children were to stay in our rooms for the duration of the visit. We were expected to read or sit quietly so as not to make our presence known. This was very disappointing to my mother's father who loved to see his grandchildren. The only time we were able to spend time with him was when he would take us fishing on his boat on Lake Sinclair. My father loved to go fishing and could not allow us not to go when my grandfather asked for all of us to come. My mother's father had a droll sense of humor and loved to use it on his grandkids. Once when we went fishing, I was watching him. He quickly put his hand in his mouth, swished something around very fast and hard in the water, and then popped it in his mouth. My face must have been quite shocked as I thought he had pulled a live fish from the water and was eating it raw (he had actually only rinsed his false teeth in the lake). Another time when I landed a particularly large Blue Gill, he kept meowing behind his hand and telling me I had caught the very first catfish from Lake St. Clair. Being the naïve little girl I was, I actually believed him.

The time of year that I felt Grandpa Edison showed his love for his three grandchildren the most was at Easter time. My father would insist on spending Easter with his mother. Every Easter evening, when we returned home from my Grandma Fischer's farm, there would be three beautifully homemade baskets with beautifully hand-painted eggs sitting on the garage floor by the back door. My Grandfather would make the drive from Detroit to Mt. Clemens, knowing we would not be home, and leave his three love tokens by our back door. It always brought tears to my eyes.

There was nothing that made my father happier than to see his children frightened. The summer I was twelve, we were visiting his mother's house, and he forced us children to take a walk with him. He was aware of a small, densely forested area that had a log with a large branch sticking up out of the middle of it that acted as a bridge over a creek. It was very difficult to cross without falling into the little creek flowing underneath it. My middle sister, my bravest sister, was the first to attempt to cross the limb. She was almost to the other end when her leg slipped off and she stepped onto a hornet's nest giving her numerous painful stings. Next my oldest sister was told to cross. Not daring to disobey my father, she started across, sobbing. My father got on the other end of the tree and began jumping up and down to make her crossing harder. When she reached the limb in the middle of the log, she sat down and was able, by holding onto the limb, to get around it and completed crossing the log to the other side. No one was yet aware of my middle sister's experience of stepping onto the hornet's nest. She had too much pride to let my father see her cry. It was finally my turn, and I was terrified. It looked like a huge drop to the creek under the log. I started across, and following my oldest sister's example, I sat down to get around the limb sticking up in the log. I then stood up and tried to finish. By now my father was jumping up and down on the tree so hard, I was unable to keep my balance and fell, catching onto the log on my way down, which left me dangling over the creek. My father started back across the tree as if to help me and grabbed my wrists. Instead of pulling me back up, he began dipping me up and down into the water below. He was enjoying himself so much that his laughing unbalanced him, he let go of me, I fell into the water, and he fell on the hornet's nest. It was then that he finally noticed what had happened to my middle sister, and he finally rushed us back to his mother's house to take care of the hornet stings. Neither his mother nor my mother asked how it happened.

A few weeks later, we went to Canada to a sand dune park. The park had mountains of sand you could walk almost a mile or so into the lake, and it would only be knee deep. My father found a part of the beach further down where the water was deep and rocky. He swam out to a rock, stood on it, and encouraged me to walk out to him. I was too young to swim at the time. I entered the water and was walking when suddenly, about fifty feet away from reaching my father, the ground dropped out from under me. I sank immediately but was able to kick myself back up to the surface. I screamed for help, but my father was laughing so hard while standing on the rock, he had tears rolling down his face. I went under again and kicked myself back up to the surface, crying out in terror. My father finally came over and put me back on firm footing.

As my sisters and I approached our teens, they became interested more in fashion and style and began to practice applying makeup and spent more time with my mother shopping. I had no interest in any of these pastimes and was just as happy washing the car or handing my father, who was an excellent mechanic, tools while he worked on the car. It was soon the accepted norm that my two sisters hung out with my mom and went shopping with her and I would stay at home and help him with projects around the house or working on the car. I had no idea of the dangerous position I was allowing myself to fall into, nor was I aware of the manipulation on his part to try to separate me from my mother and sisters.

Chapter 3

My Teen Years

I started playing the clarinet in the fifth grade and fell in love with the sound. I practiced every day and sat first chair for all my junior high concerts. For rehearsals I was placed back in the third row as the director preferred to flirt with the giggly, talkative girls during rehearsal, and I was always quiet.

By the time I turned fourteen, I had begun my monthly menstrual cycle. When I went to high school Physical Education class, I was teased by the other ninth grade Physical Education students because my father would not allow me to wear a bra. It was most embarrassing. In the summer of my fourteenth year, we spent our vacation at Happy Hank's in the upper peninsula of Michigan. It was a dude ranch, and we had a wonderful time. It was at Happy Hank's that I received my first kiss from one of the teens who were employed to lead the trail rides and be sure the patrons of the ranch had a good time. I was embarrassed and ashamed as the teen boy who chose me to focus on stuck his tongue in my mouth during the kiss, and I felt it was gross. I avoided him the rest of our stay.

That fall when I was going into High School, I soon discovered why my father had worked so hard to separate out his relationship with me in comparison to his relationship with my sisters. He ignored my oldest sister and he had her convinced she was too dumb to talk to and would amount to nothing. My second eldest sister and my father were always at odds. It was a love-hate relationship. My sister adored my father, would excel in school classes to focus his attention on her accomplishments. Her attempts to please my father only made him view her as being arrogant and pushy.

My mother joined a bowling league that played on Wednesday evenings. My father was actually quite encouraging of her getting out and even bought her a pink bubblegum bowling ball and her own set of bowling shoes. About October of my freshman year in High School, my relationship with my father changed. One Wednesday night after all three of us girls had been sent to bed at our usual 9:00 PM bedtime, my father came into my room and invited me to watch TV with him. The show we watched was the *Jonathan Winters Show*, which I came to love. It was my first introduction to adult comedy. The next Wednesday, he again told me to come and watch the show, and without hesitation, I followed him into the living room. This time he was sitting on the sofa and was wearing only a robe. He sat with his back to the arm of the sofa and invited me to sit on his lap. I was a little afraid at first but did as he told me. After watching the show for about fifteen minutes, he did something that alarmed me and that I instinctively knew was wrong. He put his hand up my pajama top and began to rub my breast and squeeze my nipples. Too scared to get off, I stayed put and watched the remainder of the show. I could feel his erection through my thin nightgown.

Since nothing further developed, I relaxed a little bit and was willing to leave my bed the following Wednesday night to watch the *Jonathan Winters Show*, which I loved by this time. I can understand why Robin Williams calls him his favorite comic. Once again he parked me on his lap, but this time, he was sitting in a normal upright position. He had me lie across his lap with my head propped up by a few pillows and the arm of the sofa, so I had a clear view of the TV. It was the first TV model in the neighborhood that was color, so it was quite a treat to be able to watch it while my sisters slept unknowingly. As I watched this time, my father uncovered my breasts and began his usual rubbing. After about fifteen minutes of this, he leaned down and began sucking and running his tongue across my nipples. Being the young lady in the throes of hormone activity at its peak, I could not prevent my body from reacting to his tongue on my nipples and began excreting more fluids from my vaginal canal. Once more I felt his erection and grew alarmed but was too ashamed at my body's reaction and afraid to stop him. He couldn't help but notice my physical reaction to his sexual advances and slowly moved his hand down across my ribs and slid it under my PJ bottoms and began stroking between my legs. In seconds I had an orgasm. I was simultaneously frightened, confused, and worried of what my mother would think of me. I knew what my father did was very wrong but was too scared to stop him. The show finished, and I went to bed.

The following Wednesday, I lay in bed in terror, knowing the time would come when he would ask me to watch TV with him. This time I said no. This did not deter him. He came into my bedroom, closed the door, and kneeled beside my bed. He went through the same routine, and once more, my body reacted as the last Wednesday. This time he stayed longer, tried again after a short time, and was able to make me have a second orgasm. I told him that if he didn't stop, I would tell my mother. Suddenly he was not so friendly and threatened to kill me if I told anyone what he was doing. He told me if I told, my mother would want a divorce, and it would be my fault for breaking up the family. As the episodes continued to happen, I tried, in childish ways, to discourage him. I would wear two pairs of pajamas, hoping to make it too difficult for him. He never said anything and also didn't let it slow him down.

During the following summer, we once more went to Hank's Dude Ranch. At first I felt safe as my parents slept in a separate room than we daughters. My sisters signed up for every trail ride available, and I preferred splashing around and looking for shells along the shoreline. One afternoon, as I was walking alone, out of sight of any other patrons, my father came up behind me. He took off his swimsuit and insisted I do the same. He entered the water up to his neck and insisted I join him. I dog paddled to him as I was a very poor swimmer. I was forced to clutch my arms around his neck with our bodies pressed together. I could feel his hard erect male organ, and I was terrified that I was about to be raped but still hung on to him for dear life as my fear of the water was even stronger. He did not penetrate me, but after some time, he allowed me to go back to shore and put my suit back on, and he did the same.

My father began looking for more and more opportunities to molest me. That summer between my ninth and tenth grade years, my father paid to have the basement finished, so it now had a bar, family room, storage room, and laundry/utilities room. He insisted I practice my clarinet in the downstairs family room and would come down when I practiced and molest me. He became more aggressive, asking me to do things to him, and I began to fight back. He tried to put a stop to this first by threatening me with an air rifle. I was terrified but did not do what he wanted me to do. He forced me to read a pornographic book with a picture of a woman bent over, her butt displayed prominently with the word "Bull's-eye" written on her butt hole and the rest of the target painted around it. It sickened me rather than aroused me. He never tried that tactic again.

One night, the following fall, when I was a sophomore in High School and my mother was once more bowling on Wednesday nights, he made me leave my bedroom and drink some awful alcoholic drink. While I drank it, fearing he would spank me if I didn't, he told me stories of his boyhood on the farm and how he and his brother used to get into cow chip fights. Suddenly everything he said was hilariously funny, and I felt quite strange. He told me to finish the drink, and when I had, I couldn't walk without falling down I blacked out at this point, and when I woke up in my bed the following morning, my eyes were bloodshot and my hair was so full of vomit it stood out about a foot from my head. I was suffering a serious headache. My father was back on the afternoon shift again and made sure he was up when I got up. He told my mother, who was shocked and horrified by my appearance, that I must have some twenty-four-hour virus and told me to go take a shower. My mother accepted his explanation without question and did nothing.

When the alcohol and the vulgar book didn't have the effect he was looking for, he tried one more thing that worked splendidly. My father had installed a new engine in our 1954 Buick and had an open offer for a job at the gas station at the head of our street anytime he wanted one. He also had a large (five-foot) canister of welding gas for his mechanical use when needed. He began using the plastic bag his shirts came from the laundry in, filling it with propane gas and holding it over my head until I would pass out. It worked for him, but I doubted he knew if it would harm me and was terrified one day he would overdo it and I would never wake up. When the bag went over my head, I would hold my breath as long as possible so as not to breathe the fumes. When I finally did take a breath, it was a pretty large one. I remember just before I would pass out all sounds seemed to echo over and over until I passed out. I began to have burns around my neck from the gas and the plastic bag wrapped around my neck.

One day when I was practicing my clarinet, my father came into the basement with the bag. He forced it over my head, and after a short time, I was passed out. I started to come out of it and could feel I was naked with a bottle inserted up my vaginal canal. My father threw a blanket over me he kept on hand to cover me up if someone came down unexpectedly. I could hear my middle sister asking my dad if I was OK. He told her I was fine, and she was to go back upstairs. She did as she had been told. As soon as the upstairs door shut, my father once more put the bag over my head. The taste of the gas would remain in my mouth for hours afterward. I would spit and spit trying to get rid of the taste. For many years, after I left home, I would gag at the smell of gasoline fumes.

When I was a senior in high school, I once more auditioned for band. My band teacher told me I played better than anyone else but would have to sit in the third chair as I still played on a plastic clarinet. I was so angry and sad. I did not want to ask my father for a wood clarinet because I knew what he would expect of me if he got me one. I was unwilling to pay the price. Apparently my high school band director called my parents and explained the situation to them as one day, about a week after I had auditioned, I came to dinner and found a new wood clarinet on my chair. Unfortunately my father picked out the cheapest wood clarinet he could find. It played worse than my plastic horn. When I brought it to school and showed it to the band director, he didn't say anything but told me to leave the clarinet with him. He then let me try some Buffet clarinets (the top of the line), and I found one with a tonal quality that I fell in love with.

A few days later, the same clarinet was sitting on my chair at the kitchen when I came out for breakfast. I was so excited. My father tried to imply that I owed him something in return for the clarinet. I stubbornly refused to allow him to molest me, so the gassing continued throughout my senior year in High School.

I kept silent because I felt responsible to keep the family together. My father said my mother would divorce him if she found out and it would hurt my sisters. He squarely placed the blame on me if I told. I gave no thought to a career as I didn't ever see an end to my private nightmare. I began babysitting as much as I possibly could because I felt much safer in a stranger's house than I did in my own. Because I was not allowed to spend any of the money I made from babysitting jobs at $.50 an hour, I had the cash to buy a brand-new car immediately after graduation.

My father also allowed me to have a boyfriend in my junior and senior years. The boy I went out with was affiliated with a Masonic group, which my father, who was a Mason, approved of. Also he assumed my boyfriend was a nerd and would be too scared to help me if I were to tell him. I saw my first indoor movie with him. I saw my first play with him. I broke it off during the middle of my senior year as I knew the relationship was not based on love. By May of my senior year, I wrote to him at the Air Force Academy where he was attending as his brother had before him. He hated the lifestyle and the hazing and ended up quitting before I graduated. He went to a local technical university. We got back together because I had found out my father was being transferred to Canfield, Ohio, to work at the new Fisher Body plant to prepare for the newest technology in engines. The four-cylinder Vega automobile was made to compete with the influx of European cars, which were much more energy efficient.

The house I had known as home all my life was sold two weeks before I was to graduate from high school. Also my oldest sister was due to get married the day after my graduation. I was not to receive, as my sisters did, a graduation party. My band teacher invited me to live with him during the week and stay with my family on weekends. My mother was quick to accept being kept busy with my sister's wedding plans; she had little or no time to spend with me.

On the weekend, my father came back to Michigan to get me to take me to Canfield to see my new home. The home was in a rich area. It was twice the home that we had had before. It took me time to be able to find my way among the maze of rooms. My father took me to meet one of his coworkers, and after having dinner at their house, he took me to a motel room where he had booked one room as the house was not ready for occupation yet. That was one of the worst nights of my life. My father forced me to sleep in the bed with him. I was allowed to wear my pajamas, but he was completely nude. I did not sleep all night terrified of what he might try to do. The following day, he had to work. While he worked, I spent my time in the bathroom being severely ill. When he came back to the motel, we left for Michigan. The following weekend was my oldest sister's wedding. I attended my graduation and stayed one more night at the mobile home of my mother's friend Mickey, where my mother had been staying for two months. I went to my sister's wedding the next evening and stayed one more night with my mother. Before leaving, I had a final date with my boyfriend, and when he asked me to marry him, I finally confessed to what had been going on between my father and I. He held me for a while, but my father sized him up right. He did nothing but say he would talk it over with his mother and get her advice. The following day, my mother and I met my father in Canfield, Ohio, and made ourselves at home in our new house. I applied to the Dana School of Music and auditioned and was accepted. My father would not allow me to stay on the campus but insisted I must stay at home. Knowing his reason why, I ended up losing interest in school and never sent in tuition.

The Labor Day after my graduation brought matters between my father and I to a head. My middle sister brought three friends over for the weekend. I had no warning when on Monday, Labor Day, my mother took me aside and informed me she was going back to Michigan to divorce my father and I was to stay with him. I panicked, I cried, I pleaded with her not to leave me alone with him, but she said she had stayed in the marriage only to make sure all of us children finished school and no longer felt obligated to continue the sham of a marriage. She told me my father was absolutely set against my going with her. She was willing to sacrifice my safety for her freedom. A few hours later, all the company was gone, and I was alone with my father, not knowing anyone in the area to go to for help. My father was extremely angry with my mother for leaving him. That night was the night I thought would be my last. He forced me to sit on his lap and then proceeded to poison my mind with stories of how he would commit suicide to pay back my bitch of a mother. He told me she had been unfaithful to him several times. He ranted and raved, and when finally I struggled to get away, he slapped me across the back of my head. I had blood pouring out of my ears and nose. He then dumped me off his lap, unconscious, and after filling a bag of plastic full of gas, he put it over my head as I was coming to.

He must have carried me into his and my mother's room. When I came to, I was very, very sore in my vaginal area. He told me to get out of his room. I waddled to my bedroom and fell asleep immediately. When I woke up the next morning, he had gone to work. I took several showers, trying to wash the touch of him off me. After I was dressed, I went into the kitchen and automatically began cleaning my blood off the kitchen floor. I was sure that if I did not get away that day, I would not live to see another. I called the boy I had been dating in Michigan, and he and his mother came and picked me up. I had little to pack. I brought my clarinet and a few clothes. There was little else I chose to bring as there was nothing but memories of childhood nightmares attached to all my belongings.

My boyfriend's mother brought us back to Michigan where I had to find out where my mother was. She had recently created a partnership with a man to be a Wedding Planner. He thought it odd that I would not know how to find my mother but told me the hotel she was staying at.

We arrived and knocked on the door. She was very upset to find me there. She knew my father would be right behind me, looking to drag me back home. I told her what had happened the night before and what had been happening for the past four years. Her first reaction was at first to deny that she knew anything about it, followed by admitting knowing it for a year as my middle sister had told her what she had seen when she caught my father molesting me in the basement that one time. She admitted knowing it had to be true because my father had an adopted sister who was a teenager who told my mother that my father had molested her after my mother was married to my father. My mother told me she had too many problems to work out to take care of me too. She suggested I stay with my oldest sister who was living in a very tiny apartment above her in-laws' garage.

My oldest sister's marriage was already beginning to unravel as her husband was both an alcoholic and on drugs. Both worked during the day. The next day, I was alone in the apartment when my father called. He told me to stay where I was, and he was coming to get me and take me back to Ohio to live with him. I hung up in terror and called my mother who would not help me. I then called my now-fiancé's mother and asked for her help once again. She found me a place to stay with some wonderful people who were very kind to me. They helped me find a job as a teacher's aide in a summer school for inner-city children. I stayed at their home for about a week and later ended up moving into my fiancé's house. My fiancé, Joseph, was still in college and wasn't expected to graduate for a couple of years. But we were engaged anyway. I visited my band teacher during the next few days. I discovered he had always thought there was something not right about my parents. They never came to any of my band concerts, and my mother was always afraid to speak to him. He had somehow twisted my Dad's arm to get me my clarinet.

He helped me find my first full-time job as a bookkeeper at a bank. I still did not know how to drive but managed to buy, with my babysitting earnings, a new Vega with automatic transmission. I arranged a day when I could pick up the car at my father's house while he wasn't there. By this time, he had given up on forcing me back to live with him, so I was able to come get the Vega I had arranged to pay for while he was not home. I drove it back to Detroit, Michigan. After a few months of at-the-wheel training, I took and passed my driver's test. For the next year, I worked full time at the bank. After a few months, when I was feeling a little more secure, I told my fiancé I would like to move out of his mother's home and get my own place. He became very agitated and told me I only agreed to be engaged to him to get away from my father. It was true, but to hear it said made me feel very guilty, so I quickly backed down. We were married in March of 1973. I worked sixty-hour weeks and only had Sundays free for housekeeping, shopping, and other miscellaneous errands. My new husband, Joseph, had his mother over every Sunday to take us out for dinner as a treat.

I became pregnant while on the pill and needed to have some time alone. I requested my husband to ask his mother to cut her visits down to once every two weeks. He patiently explained to me that we were her only family, and it was too much of a change for her and would cause her pain. Finally in November of that year (1974), I put my foot down and told her myself. She became very hurt and said she wouldn't bother us anymore. I found dealing with her exasperating, almost as bad as her son.

When we first started our life as a married couple in a mobile home his mother had bought for us, I asked Josh to empty the garbage. He said he had never done so before and had no idea how it was done. I began to explain to Josh where to find the plastic garbage bags. Deciding it would be easier to just do it myself, I emptied the trash and took responsibility for all the housework from then on.

Our first son, Jeremy Joseph, arrived the day after Christmas. I could no longer work, so Joseph began working in a bank while he finished the last year of his degree in Computer Programming. He was a brilliant mathematician, but had poor social skills. He didn't brush his teeth, so I was in the position of acting as his surrogate mother, reminding him when to bathe, brush his teeth, etc. I was not familiar with "normal" so did not find fault with him, but I was very frustrated all the time.

After he graduated in the spring, Joseph sent resumes all over the country at a time of high unemployment, with gas prices raised to over $1 per gallon, and record high interest rates. He received only one positive reply, and it would mean moving out of Michigan. I told him he should take the position, which he did. I now had to deal with his older brother who was a lifetime air force military person. He called and told me how selfish I was to take his mother's only son out of the area. I responded that he should have thought of that possibility himself when he chose his career, which has taken him all over the world. I told him his mother was stronger than he gave her credit for and she had friends and other relatives in the area to help her if the need ever arose.

So after a month, we packed up our items, taking only the rocking chair with us for furniture, and headed to Eagan, Minnesota, where Unisys was located. We rented an apartment near his workplace. It was a lonely winter for me, but when spring came, I met a woman who would become a mentor for me in my early twenties.

Meanwhile, many factors were combining to leave me open to Parkinsonism. I was exposed quite heavily to the gas used by welders. I was exposed to extreme stress at the hands of my father and my new husband and his family, and unknown to me, I had two mutations of my Parkin2 gene, making me much more likely to develop Parkinsonism. It was only a matter of time before symptoms developed.

Chapter 4

My Twenties

I was in the laundry room washing another load of diapers in the apartment building when I heard the door open behind me and a heavy five-foot, middle-aged woman with short blond hair popped her head in the door. "Everyone must be doing laundry today. The downstairs one is busy too. Of course the one downstairs has been stopped for over an hour and two other baskets of dirty laundry are piled up behind it, waiting to be washed. I wish they would just put their clean clothes into the dryer and start their next load." I promised to come down to her apartment and let her know the machine would be available when my load was done. A half hour later, I was back to the laundry room on my floor and waited the final few minutes for the load to stop spinning. I then placed the freshly cleaned diapers into the dryer, inserted the coins needed to dry them, and went back to my apartment to collect Jeremy who had just woken from his afternoon nap. He was beginning his second year of life and enjoyed walking and scooting up and down the stairs. I went down the stairs with Jeremy scooting along behind me. I waited for him to catch up and opened the heavy metal first-floor door. I held his hand as he waddled down the hall next to me and knocked on the woman's door to let her know the washing machine was available. She opened her apartment door and gratefully heard my news. She had two children. One, a boy named Justin, was almost five, and Marie was almost exactly Jeremy's age. I agreed to stay and watch her children while she went up to the laundry to start her loads.

Justin and Marie were active preschoolers. It was Jeremy's first interaction with children his own age. Marie was a headstrong young infant and did not want to share her toys with the new little intruder. They began a quarrel immediately and kept pulling the toy in question back and forth between them. I had no idea how to resolve the insurrection when I heard the apartment door slam. Tammy, as it turned out her name was, immediately began, without hesitation, to yell quite loudly at Marie and told her she would have to share her toys. Marie immediately released the toy, and Jeremy promptly sat down abruptly on his butt, toy in hand. Marie found another more suitable toy that she actually wanted anyway and the three preschool children played quietly together

I learned that her full name was Tammy Peterson. She originally was from upper Michigan where she met Paul, her husband, while she was getting a master's degree. She didn't seem to mind that I did not talk about myself too much and rattled on and on about herself and her family. Josh was going to be home soon, and the laundry I had transferred to the drier was dry. I pulled Jeremy up from his play and said my good-byes. Jeremy willingly followed me out the door and scooted his way back up the stairs where we went to the laundry room and collected our clean diapers. Then we went back to the apartment where Jeremy started pushing around his favorite toy, a popcorn pusher that popped little balls up and down as he pushed it from room to room on the carpet. I finished folding the diapers and put them under the changing table and then began cooking dinner. Josh and I had now gotten into a routine. He came home, had dinner, watched TV, and went to bed. He left all the cleanup and baby watching to me.

In the spring, when the children came out of the buildings to play on the playground equipment, all the mothers came out too, including Tammy. I naturally said hi to her first because outside of Josh, I knew no one else in Minnesota. Tammy was the best friend and mentor one could ever wish for. She became my chosen mother, sister, friend, and confidant.

Paul, Tammy's husband, was totally the opposite of Josh. When he came home from work, he participated in cleaning up the kitchen after meals, played with his children, and put them to bed right alongside Tammy. He was as easy to talk to as Tammy was. I had always been shy around men but not with Paul. When the two of them had a disagreement, they were both not shy about making their views known. They had no trouble yelling at each other when angry. Five minutes later, you would never expect they disagreed on anything. Justin, the oldest child, followed Paul everywhere he would go. He walked just like his dad, with a farmers' stance.

Tammy and Marie were both look-alikes. Both were blond and pretty. Marie grew up to become a Police Officer. I never heard what Justin became. The entire eleven months that we lived in the apartment complex, I spent every waking moment to learn how to parent from this couple. Paul and Tammy are devoutly Catholic and are very active in their church.

After living in the apartments for eleven months, Josh and I bought a small townhouse in Apple Valley. Our realtor was either inexperienced or not detail oriented as the townhouse had been a rental property before we bought it. We did not know that this would be significant. This classified the following year as non-homestead taxes. We bought the house with an adjustable rate mortgage when the interest was in the two-figure range. The first year we had no problem making the payments. For a time, Paul and Tammy's family lived with us while they closed on a house they had bought in Lonsdale. They could not sign a year lease for an apartment and stayed for just two weeks. After they moved away, I grew very lonely. I tried to sell Avon products door-to-door in an effort to make a friend, but most of the doors were not opened when I knocked because both parents worked.

There was a set of apartments across the street from where we lived. I tried there. There was already a woman who sold Jenny Kay products and was she ever upset that I came on her turf with Avon. She did her best to convince me to switch to selling Jenny Kay products instead, but they required you to host parties and demonstrate their products. I had no one to invite to these parties, so I just gave up trying to sell any beauty products.

The following year was a desperate time for Josh and I financially. Our first rise in our adjustable rate mortgage kicked in as well as the non-homestead taxes. Our savings slowly were dwindling down to nothing. I had a miscarriage in the fifth month of a pregnancy on Easter day. I was soon very depressed. Josh was offered an opportunity to work on a site in Tampa, Florida, which also meant better pay with a daily per-diem. We jumped at the chance. We were able to sell the townhouse quickly and moved out with a savings balance of $0. Had we waited any longer, we would have had to foreclose on our mortgage. Paul and Tammy came to help us pack up the Ryder rental truck we rented to make the move. Josh had rented a manual transmission, which neither of us had any experience driving because it was cheaper than an automatic, and he didn't know there was a difference.

After the truck was loaded, Paul took me into the garage. He told me I had to be the man in the house because he knew Josh would not have the courage to try to learn what was needed to drive a manual transmission truck. He taught me how to work the transmission and clutch together. After making me repeat back his instructions, he and Tammy headed for home, and we spent the last night in our townhouse.

Bright and early the next morning, Josh packed up my Vega (he had also bought a Vega GT model when I bought mine but blew out his transmission in two years, so my Vega was our only car.) He placed Jeremy in his child seat in the back. Jeremy always immediately fell asleep in the car.

With some grinding of the truck transmission (after all I had never driven a stick shift before), I had my first experience of running the truck through the gears without losing the power of the engine. It was a long, tiring drive. I followed Josh and Jeremy as Josh was an excellent navigator. After a couple of days driving the truck, I was actually beginning to enjoy myself. Men, unaccustomed to seeing a young woman in the driver's seat of a large truck, honked and gave me the thumbs-up sign. Soon we hit the mountains in the southeastern states. I began seeing "runaway truck ramps," which gave me the heebie-jeebies. I threw the truck into third gear and crept down the mountains as cautiously as I was able. Josh was out of my sight most of the time because he could not go slow enough to stay back with me. I finally made it to the bottom of the mountains though and saw that he had pulled along the side of the interstate to wait for me. I was getting low on gas at this point, so we pulled into the first available gas station.

I am afraid I scared the owner of the station out of his wits. I pulled the truck up to an available pump. Suddenly the station owner was running out the door of the station, waving his hands wildly and pointing up. He was terrified my truck would not fit under the canopy covering the pumps. I was very lucky as there was about six inches to spare. It did teach me a valuable lesson, and from that point on, we only stopped at truck stops for gas.

We reached Tampa uneventfully and unloaded the truck into the house, our first time living in one of our own and turned in the truck unharmed. I found out shortly after we moved in that I was expecting my third baby. The house was a typical Florida house. It had no basement, one window air conditioner that did not work well, and the one space heater was placed in the hallway to heat the entire home

It was interesting in Tampa/St. Petersburg. The bridges all had pelicans on the tops of the lights. While living there, we had the opportunity to visit places such as Busch Gardens, Disney World, and the Kennedy Space Center. Josh and I could finally eat out on occasion. One of my favorite memories is of a German restaurant in St. Petersburg. The tables were all on the sides of the two-story building. In the center was a trampoline on which acrobats were continuously performing their complicated shows. There were strolling tuba players who would play by your table in return for whatever change you would throw into the bells of their sousaphone. Jeremy loved to try throwing the quarters we gave him into the bell of the horns. He wasn't very good at it, but was very enthusiastic.

Jeremy was three and still not consistent about using the potty and did not talk. I had always sensed something was wrong with his growth. He screamed constantly in the hospital when he was born, upsetting all the babies, so the nurses tried to keep him in my room with me as much as possible. He cried most of the time and had to be bottle-fed because of his impatience with waiting for my milk to drop from my milk ducts. The only time he seemed to be happy was when I walked him in a stroller, swung him in a swing, or when he was riding in the car. At three years of age, he still was not sleeping through the night, would scream anytime he went shopping with us, and I was tired most of the time.

Being in Florida where the heat and humidity were up in the hundreds with a little air conditioner that didn't even cool the living room and, to top it off, being seven months pregnant did not make me a pleasant person to be around. I was crabby all the time. Nothing made me happy. I wanted to go home to Minnesota where it was cool. Josh was upset with me, for good cause, as I was a mean-spirited person to spend time with. Nothing he did would satisfy me. Shortly before he was done with his project and we could go back home to Minnesota, I went into labor. Josh had all the nursing attention as he was out in the waiting room vomiting with a case of the flu. Meanwhile I endured the labor by myself in the birthing room. When the nurses saw I was fully dilated, they called the doctor who delivered me of a second baby boy whom we named James Steve. Where Jeremy had always screamed, James was very calm. He, like Jeremy, was unable to breast-feed. James had lactose intolerance, and soy formula became his drink of the day.

A week before we were to leave for Minnesota, I took James and Jeremy to a pediatrician for James's first checkup. The pediatrician watched Jeremy run screaming around his office, picking up all the medical instruments and examining them carefully. As the doctor examined James, I attempted to keep Jeremy still. After the doctor was done examining James, he turned and said to me, "No wonder you always look so tired. Have you had Jeremy evaluated for any emotional or mental problems?" I could have kissed him. I had been to about eight psychologists already, seven for opinions on Jeremy's behavior, and had been told he was a little behind for his age but not enough to cause worry. I then scheduled an appointment for myself and told the psychologist I had to be a bad mother because of Jeremy's crying all the time.

James's pediatrician set me up with an appointment with the Florida children's evaluation center for the next day. They diagnosed

Jeremy within a few minutes of observation as mentally disturbed and retarded. I felt their diagnosis was wrong. Jeremy was not retarded as he was already able to read. I had read to him and taught him his ABCs, and he was able to count to twenty. The day following, Jeremy was vomiting constantly and could not keep food or liquids down. After two days of this, I took him to James's pediatrician who hospitalized him for dehydration. Jeremy was in the hospital for two days. I stayed with him for every visiting hour allowed. Meanwhile James also began vomiting and becoming dehydrated. Jeremy was sent home, and James took his place in the hospital. We were supposed to be leaving for Minnesota in two days. We had arranged to have our belongings moved by a professional moving company this time and had booked tickets on the Amtrak Auto train to Maryland, from where we planned to drive through Ohio, to visit my dad, and Michigan to visit with Joseph's mother and my mother and sisters.

James was released the day we boarded the Amtrak train. He slept all day, and Jeremy was kept fascinated by looking out the window at the mostly manufacturing towns we passed through. We had dinner, and then we were to sleep in coach. James had slept just about the whole day, so he was pretty hungry during the night. He woke up every two hours during the night for feedings. I could hear several groans throughout our car. I felt no sympathy after what I had been through that week and was glad of the company while I fed him. The following morning, we reached Maryland and, by nighttime, were at my father's house. I still hadn't dealt with my feelings about my father and kept them bottled up inside me in an effort to keep the family together. I was ever watchful of my children and would immediately put a stop to any bullying he tried. Mealtimes were especially worrisome. Jeremy was a very fussy eater, and my father tried to force him to eat things Jeremy didn't like. My father would stop when I told him to. My father was remarried now to a woman named Helen. Helen's first marriage had been to an abusive alcoholic, so it was a perfect match.

In the morning, we made our way to Michigan where we stayed with Josh's mother in our old mobile home. My mother and sisters came to visit us at the mobile home. My oldest sister had a baby named Thomas whom I made quite a fuss over. Her marriage had ended before his birth, and she was raising him on her own. I greeted my mother and other sister but generally focused on the new baby. My middle sister told me I looked fat. Apparently my mother felt I was rude for not giving her more attention because just before Josh and I were to go back to Minnesota, I got a call from my oldest sister dressing me down for not giving my mother enough attention. This visit made me angry toward my whole family. No matter how hard I tried I could never satisfy any of them.

I was very relieved to get back to Minnesota. Josh had gone back shortly before the whole family to find us a place to live. He had picked out a rental townhouse of about five floors. The basement had the laundry. The second level was the garage; the third level was the kitchen, dining room, and living room. The fourth level had two bedrooms for the children and a full bathroom, and the fifth level had a massive master bedroom with its own quarter bath. This is where we were living when I took Jeremy around for his first Halloween Trick or Treat. Jeremy ended up eating too much candy and was violently ill that night. I felt very guilty for allowing him to overdo it.

The next day, I called the county social services department and asked to have an evaluation done for Jeremy to see if he could qualify for some type of helpful intervention. He was evaluated and determined to have a mild form of brain damage in the auditory processing part of his brain. He began going to a full day program to try to integrate him and correct some of his social skills. I noticed a difference in his behavior immediately. He loved his teacher, Nancy, who worked with him to follow routines, stay on tasks, and interact with other children appropriately. Jeremy would only play with a group of children if he were in charge. If angry, he would go off by himself and try to hit anyone who tried to redirect his behavior.

For the next year, I found life to be a lot less complicated and stressed. I enjoyed James. He was a sweet baby and had a wonderful sense of fun. He loved to play peekaboo and loved to be read to. We could play imaginative games. His favorite thing to do was to help me cook in the kitchen. Like Jeremy, James was also a fussy eater. James and Jeremy got on well as children because James was perfectly happy to let Jeremy lead the play. We once more bought a townhouse in a city called Inver Grove Heights.

Shortly after we moved there, my father came for a visit with his new wife. I carefully watched his interaction with the children and found him playing the same games with them that he used to do to us girls when we were young. Jeremy hated to be controlled in any way and fought back, but James was easygoing and didn't understand what my father was doing. After they left, I began to feel anger building in me. I was angry at my sisters for the treatment I had received on my visit when coming back to Minnesota. I was angry with my mother for playing her little game of martyr to complain of my behavior to my oldest sister and make her feel responsible to protect my mother's feelings. And most of all, I was angry at my father for being allowed to keep his dirty little secret of what he had done to me without receiving any repercussion for his vile behavior. I began to go to see a social worker to discover how to deal with my intense anger over what had happened to me nearly six years prior. The social worker asked me if I was getting anything out of the current relationship with my father, and I promptly answered no. "Then why do you continue to allow him in your life?" Thinking it over for three or four days, I finally decided he was no father to me to begin with. I also did not want to worry about my children every time he came to visit. So I called him and told him no more visits or letters. I no longer chose to allow him in my life. He has so far honored my request. According to both of my sisters and mother, his new wife, Helen, has no idea why I cut him out in the first place.

When James was eighteen months old, I became pregnant once more. By now, my marriage was not doing too well as I was tired all the time. We had planned on having two children, and the third pregnancy came as a surprise. A very big surprise as I found out on the day I gave birth to a ten-pound one-ounce baby boy we named Jared Paul. Shortly afterward, I had my tubes tied as I did not want more children and Josh did not want to have the necessary surgery. Jared was different from the other two. He was a hearty eater and was my first and only breast-fed baby. No fickle feeding habits for this guy. By the time he was one, he was a little dynamo. He loved anything to do with Garfield and would sleep surrounded by about ten stuffed Garfield cats and one Ollie dog. He was all boy. He stuffed toads in his pockets. The only thing I ever saw him fear as a baby was an Ernie doll that talked. Whenever he saw the Ernie doll, he would run screaming from the room.

The summer Jeremy was to start third grade and James was to start Kindergarten, we moved to our house in Lakeville. It was a perfect house as far as I could tell. It had three bedrooms for the children and a master bedroom for us. It also had a huge backyard totally fenced in. We bought a swing set for the boys and settled in. The basement was finished off with a large family room, which was a playroom for the kids. There was a lake in front of the house and a pond behind the house. We bought our first and only dog, Brett, a Brittany Spaniel, who was wonderful with the kids and didn't chase our cat. I would walk him every day. I especially loved to walk him at night and watch the fireflies.

We still only had one car, my old Chevy Vega, and it was getting expensive to maintain. We decided to buy a larger car and decided on a Buick. It was a midsize car and fit all of the growing family. Josh took the only car to work.

One day, I noticed a church up the road was having a summer Bible class. I pulled the three children up the hill to the church in their red wagon and noticed I had one heck of a stitch in my right side. I managed to make it home and lie down on the couch. The pain was getting much worse, and I wasn't sure if I would be able to climb back up the hill to get the children from Bible Summer Class.

I called Josh at work but reached a secretary who said she would leave him a message. When it was approaching twelve noon, when the Bible Study was done, I still hadn't heard from Josh. I dragged myself off the couch, pulled the wagon up the hill, picked up the three children and pulled them back home. I was in agony by that time and could not get lunch for the boys. Fortunately, the church had given them a snack just before they had come home.

It was four hours after I had given the secretary the message before Josh finally called back. I told him I had to go to the doctor's immediately, but he had about a half-hour drive, which seemed like forever as the pain intensified. He came home to take me to the doctor. As soon as I was seen, I was rushed to the hospital, and my appendix was removed. The surgeon who removed it said he was sure it would rupture before he got it out.

Time went fast, and before I was ready, Jared entered Kindergarten, and I was home alone for a half a day. I was quite lonely. We received a mailing from a local community college that was looking for musicians to play in band class. I took my old clarinet out of the closet and began practicing. I signed up and went on Monday evenings from 6:30 to 9:30 PM. The first time I went, there were seventeen clarinet players: eight players on first clarinet, eight players on second clarinet, and myself on third clarinet. The director announced that after the first concert, there would be chair auditions.

The week after the concert, the clarinet section only had six members. After the auditions, I was ranked second, and the following year, the person who ranked first dropped out of the band, so I was now the first chair player. I also began to take clarinet lessons from a man I consider to be the best teacher ever, Claude Mercer. My playing improved tremendously. I found that people in the band actually liked me and started to develop friends outside of the family.

When I was to play my first concert as first chair, my husband decided to come and bring the three children. It was in December, and he was scheduled to take a flight out of town about two hours after the concert was over. During the first half of the concert, a blizzard hit the twin cities. Josh, concerned that he would miss his plane, told me at intermission he was taking a cab to the airport and that I would be responsible to get the children home after the concert.

The concert went well. When I took the children out to the car, visibility was only about twenty feet. It was a fairly long drive home on winding roads. We almost made it, but the car stalled out about a half mile from home, so I had to carry two children, one was able to walk, and carry my clarinet too. It was the coldest I have ever felt. We made it home and got into the house. My husband called to see how things had gone and spent much time telling me how much different the weather was in Florida, his work destination. When I told him I had to leave the car alongside the road, he became very upset and told me I had to find a way to get the car home in the garage where it would be safe. I tried to reason with him by explaining how we had barely made it home. He was quite angry to have our new Buick on the street, but there was nothing he could do from there, and I felt I could do nothing from home.

The next day, I shoveled out our driveway and walked back to where I had left the car with a shovel in hand. I shoveled out the car, pulled as much snow out of the exhaust pipe, and the car started up immediately. I drove it home and parked it in the garage.

The following January, I decided to try to get my bachelors degree. I wasn't quite sure what I wanted one in, so I found out what the basic core classes were at the school I attended to get a liberal arts degree and began with English and speech classes. To my amazement, I got an A in both classes. Although I had worked in the early part of our marriage sixty-hour shifts to help Josh get through school, he refused to help or make any changes in his lifestyle to help me find time to study. We tried marital counseling, but he would attempt to change for one or two weeks and then slip into old habits.

Meanwhile, I was working day and night to keep the house clean (Josh did not do any outdoor or indoor work), and it took almost a whole day just to mow the grass. After the first semester of college, I was exhausted, and I went into a clinical depression. I moved to the basement bedroom and spent day and night in the dark. I didn't sleep, lost thirty pounds in a month and was basically committing suicide in a passive way. Josh just ignored my behavior, started buying pizza or Kentucky Fried Chicken for the kid's dinner. He never once approached the downstairs bedroom to see if I was OK. I cried day and night. When I finally called First Call for Help, I was referred to a social worker. I made and kept the appointment. I was immediately put on antidepressant medication. After talking to the social worker, I finally made the decision to leave my marriage of eleven years.

When I told Josh I wanted a divorce, he became very upset. I also lost the respect and connection with Tammy and Paul. Being very devout Catholics, they could not condone my decision to divorce Joseph. He didn't cope well with change, and change was what I needed to survive. I promised not to take the children away or to fight over the house. I wanted nothing from him but out. I did need a car and promised to find the least expensive one I could. I found a car just a few miles from home at a dealership for under $2,000. The car was a stick shift Dodge Omni. I found a job working for the credit department for a Hearing Aid Manufacturer. I moved in with a band member friend, and the marriage ended quite amicably. My husband and I both used the same attorney, and I signed a quitclaim deed to the house as my share of the child custody expenses. The divorce was finalized on January 2, 1986. I had just begun to live independently at the age of thirty-two. I didn't know it, but I now had only two years to make up for my lost childhood before my senior citizen symptoms were to set in.

Chapter 5

The Thirtieth to Thirty-fifth Year

I moved in with a friend from my music contacts, Laurence Trestle. We both played in the concert band at the community college. He played baritone. He had a house on Riverside Drive in Burnsville. It was in the Walden development, and he was a new realtor and was having trouble making his payments. I usually made the house payment from my earnings as a secretary, and he covered what was left. We lived mostly on vegetables and rice. I was very happy. I was hired by the Chimera Theatre group as a pit musician and waited tables at a Bonanza Steak restaurant. In the little spare time I had, I finished my liberal arts degree. I also loved to take walks. I missed my children desperately and saw them as much as I was able. I went to all of their Parent-Teacher Conferences, their concerts, and whatever scouting events they were involved in as well as managing to see them every weekend. My oldest son, Jeremy was the angriest and would have nothing to do with me. It was understandable; he and I had been the closest, and he, like his father, was resistant to change. Looking back, I wish I had insisted Josh get him some social help.

One night, when Jesse and I were watching TV, he said, "Why are you shaking your foot so much?" I glanced down at the offending foot and answered, "Nervous habit I guess." I thought no more of it as it never consciously bothered me. Shortly after, Jesse decided he no longer wanted to stay in the United States and wanted to live in China. He had been taking a class in speaking Chinese at the University of Minnesota, so he helped me find an affordable apartment and, shortly after, moved to China where he is now the only American farmer of vegetables living there. When President Clinton went to China, he met Jesse. Jesse had married and seemed happy with his new life in China.

At our Christmas concert that winter, when I was thirty-three, the director had asked the drummer from his jazz band, Steve Wood, if he could help out the concert band for the concert as we were short of drummers. His father, Amos Wood, was a longtime friend and member in the trombone section. Steve made a joke at the band director's expense, but the director, being Puerto Rican, did not understand the English play on words and kept right on giving the band order of the music. I thought Steve's play on words was hilarious and laughed. My laughter caught his ear, and after the concert, he casually mentioned going out sometime. After checking him out with both his father and with his former boss, the owner of a music store who played in the trumpet section, I attended a jazz band concert, and we set up a date. I wasn't searching for romance. I was happier than I had ever been in my life, knowing I was capable of living on my own (relatively speaking, I needed to have a roommate to financially afford it) and was enjoying college as well as stretching my ability to learn different life philosophies. At that time, I was reading a lot of Emerson and Ayn Rand, having already read Socrates, Aristotle, and Plato. Through counseling, I had learned I had life choices I could make and shouldn't let others direct my life by playing on my emotion of guilt.

Even though I wasn't looking for romance, just a new friend who I could do things with, Steve and I amazingly hit it off right away on our first date. You could not find two people more opposite yet more alike. Steve was a hard worker, who knew what he wanted from life. Steve was, in my eyes, a daredevil who would try just about anything if it did not interfere with what he believed was morally right. Like me, he was an avid believer in freedom to make your choices. Sometimes they were wrong choices, but it was your right to make them. Steve made our first date. When he arrived to pick me up, I had just opened the letter I had been hoping for: permission to enter the College of St. Catherine weekend college program. I shared my news with him. We then went out to his car. The inside of the car was a mess. Since I wasn't looking for romance, I overlooked it, and we went to a place called the Emporium of Jazz. I had hardly ever danced in my life, but he spent the whole night trying to teach me how to waltz, polka, and fox-trot, but I am afraid I was a poor student. But I am a good listener, and what he needed at that time was someone who could listen.

He had just gotten back from France via Denmark, where he had spent a year trying to make his second marriage work, but it takes two to try, and he was unable to do it alone. It sounded like he really loved his ex-wife and was bitterly hurt when he came home from work one day to find a strange man in their bed. His ex-wife's name was Lonnie. Apparently they had met in a Danish bar when he was on tour in Europe with a band. When he got home, they spent hours on the phone together, and based on these phone calls, Steve decided he was in love with Lonnie and proposed to her on the phone. She accepted and, with her uninvited younger sister, in tow came to the States. Steve and his family greeted them warmly, and she and her sister were welcomed to the Wood household.

A short while later, they were married by the justice of the peace. Lonnie also had a child from a previous marriage. Eventually Lonnie declared she was unhappy living in the States and convinced Steve that Denmark was a better country to raise a family. Steve informed his family that he and Lonnie were moving back to Denmark. Everyone in the family thought it was a mistake but, knowing they could not talk Steve out of something once his mind was made up, supported his decision.

Steve, Lonnie, and baby moved to Denmark and lived with her mother (Lonnie's parents had been divorced for quite some time) until Steve could take Danish language lessons and find himself a job. His language teacher became a part of Steve's extended family, and they developed a close relationship. Meanwhile, Lonnie and her mother spent most evenings playing bingo, using up their government-subsidized monthly income. Steve found his first job at last, delivering newspapers. This required much stair-climbing as the town was built into a hill and the housing was mostly apartments. Since Steve could not afford to buy much food, and with all the fresh air and exercise he was getting, he was in the best health he had ever been. He attempted to break into the music job market, hoping to get back into jazz drumming. He was finally accepted by one musical group who had the ear to know talent when they heard it. Steve's understanding of the Danish language was a barrier for him.

One day, the leader of the group went into a tirade and fired the whole group. Steve didn't quite understand the source of the band leader's anger but packed up his drums and headed home. This same day is the time he discovered a man in bed with his wife, and Lonnie showed no remorse. Steve quit his job as a newspaper delivery person and began working as a carriage driver in a deer park to try to earn the money to fly back home. He visited frequently with his language teacher at his teacher's home. He also maintained a friendship with Lonnie's former husband, Vic, the father of her child. Lonnie reconsidered and told Steve she was pregnant, and the baby was his. Steve, being no fool, could count how many months back it had been since he had known her in that way, and it didn't work out. It took a year to receive the divorce decree. Steve then contacted the Danish government and demanded a flight back to the States.

He talked about Lonnie so much in those first six months we dated that I was beginning to think he would never get over her. But eventually, as we came to know each other better, I realized that the breakup was so hard for him to comprehend not emotionally as it was intellectually. He kept going over and over in his head, trying to understand how it could have happened from his viewpoint without taking into account Lonnie's part in the marriage. He had tried to be the perfect husband and father and still the marriage didn't work.

Eventually he stopped trying to relive the past and began living in the here and now on our new relationship. Steve and I moved in together at Sibley Manner as I was fed up with my roommate at the dorm, and he wanted to move out of his parent's house. After all, he was thirty-seven years old. So we shacked up at the same apartments his parents had lived at when they were beginning their marriage together. The first year went very well. I was busy with my jobs, shows, and school, and Steve was busy with his new job, interpreter for the deaf, playing gigs, and helping me with my homework. He was very patient and a much better tutor than my former husband had been. My former husband's response to my questions about Mathematics was an exasperated "Everyone knows that," leaving me embarrassed and ashamed to be the one person in the world who didn't. Steve was frustrated by my prickly attitude toward learning, but eventually he came to understand that I was sure I was stupid because I didn't know the basic Mathematical rules. He also tried to help me with my French Class because I genuinely wanted to learn the language so I could travel to France one day and be able to speak their language. I spent hours and hours listening to tapes, mimicking what I thought I was hearing, learning their exceptions and was unable to pass the first chapter by the middle of the semester. The

French teacher, knowing how hard I was trying, talked the Dean of Studies into waving the requirement of a language for graduation.

Steve and I used to try to walk every day. One day he asked me why I never swung my right arm. I explained it was just the way I had always been. Steve said he could recognize me from a great distance because of my peculiar gait. I never thought anything of it. After we had been living together about a year, I changed jobs. I worked for the Minnesota Housing Finance Agency as a student worker. The pay was much better, and I loved the work and the people I worked with. Steve and I moved out of Sibley Manor into an apartment in West St. Paul as the Sibley apartments were becoming infested by roaches and the person in the apartment directly above us had been mugged.

I was getting close to completing my requirements to graduate, and Steve and I had been living together for two years. We had several fights during that time because I was more controlling, and Steve was very loose. He didn't call if he went out after playing a gig; he was constantly making plans without consulting me and frequently made large purchases without talking it over with me. But I was tired of shacking up and felt ready to make a commitment. I asked Steve if he was interested in getting married, and he answered with a firm no. I said, "OK, I will move out tomorrow then because I am prepared to make a commitment, and if you are not interested, I am wasting my time in this relationship." I think it took Steve aback that I was so matter-of-fact about our situation, and he knew I was serious. The next morning, he changed his mind and agreed he too was ready to commit. We had a lovely ceremony by the justice of the peace at his parent's house.

His mentor and friend, Dean, and his wife, Sharon Sampson, were kind and set us up to stay at a lodge in Northern Minnesota called Naniboujou Lodge. My sister-in-law-to-be made my flowers and acted as photographer and Steve's younger brother, Mark, was best man and his older sister, Kris, was my maid of honor. On August 18, 1990, Steve and I became man and wife.

Our first year of marriage tested us in just about every area of stress that there is. A few months after our marriage, my ex-husband, Josh, said he would be out of town that week and asked if we would we watch the children. We agreed but wanted to watch them at our apartment rather than his house. Josh had already left for the flight by the time Steve and I arrived to pick up the children. Jared and James, accustomed to staying with Steve and myself, were ready. Jeremy, on the other hand, was determined not to leave. He decided he was old enough to stay on his own at home. I insisted he had to come with us as it was what his father wished. He said no. I went into his room and began to pack a bag for him, and he accused me of child abuse and pushed me out the door. He then slammed the door and tried to hold it shut. I won the fight over the door and, when it was opened, began to pack some clothes for him again. Jeremy became quite aggressive and began scratching and hitting me. Steve chose to intervene at this point and held Jeremy against the floor while I continued to pack some things. Jeremy was very thin and wiry and was able to squirm out of Steve's grasp. Jeremy began beating Steve with a walking stick and screaming that Steve was abusing him and I should call the police. I did call the police, not because I felt Steve was abusing Jeremy, but because Jeremy was totally out of control.

The behavior he was displaying now had always gotten him what he wanted time and time again. As we waited for the police to arrive, I checked Steve's back where Jeremy had struck him with the stick. It was badly bruised. Jeremy didn't have a mark on him. His two younger brothers sat wide-eyed on the sofa. When the police arrived, they summed up the situation, and to Jeremy's astonishment, he was handcuffed and taken to the police car.

I called his father that evening to let him know what was going on. My feelings were mixed about the situation. I loved Jeremy dearly. I could remember how the children at the bus stop would bully him constantly by chasing him away from the bus stop area. Jeremy would trudge with his backpack to the other bus stop at the other end of the street and be treated the same way. I knew if I went out and yelled at the kids, it would only give them more reason to bully him more. I tried calling both the school; they referred me to the bus garage and the bus garage who said unless something was happening while the children were on the bus, there was nothing they could do. I understood why he behaved as he did but had no power to change his situation.

Jeremy was placed in foster homes until a date could be set up in the court system to deal with his case. The judge was quite firm with him and explained to Jeremy that as long as he was under eighteen years of age, he was under his parent's jurisdiction and had to be obedient. The judge asked Jeremy if he would prefer to live in foster care for the rest of his youth or if he would like to live with Steve and I. Going back to his father's house was not an option. Jeremy reluctantly agreed to stay at Steve's and my house. Joseph was quite happy about this decision because Jeremy was feared by his brothers.

Steve, surprisingly, was also agreeable to the idea. It was a challenge he looked forward to facing as he had always been frustrated at my declining to interfere with how Joseph chose to father the children. Steve immediately began to draw up a schedule of what was allowed and what wasn't allowed in our house. Jeremy was outraged at being treated as an infant and ran away to his father's house. He only knew how to get there by freeway, so it didn't take long for us to find him. We brought him back home and told him the judge would put him in foster care for the rest of his life if he didn't comply with the court order. The pressure on both Steve and I was extreme. I found a program offered by the YMCA that would give us a breather and help Jeremy at the same time. It was a lifesaver. Jeremy went kayaking with other difficult youngsters under the supervision of a camp councilor. The trip was probably the single most important adventure that helped Jeremy to mature and learn to cooperate with others. He came back a changed teenager. When he had a relapse back to his prior behavior, I had discovered that if I took off his door to his room for a day, it would remind him who was putting a roof over his head and food in his belly, and he would be cooperative again.

In September when Jeremy started up school, he was able to start with a clean slate as it was a different school district and no one was aware that he had been bullied at his other district. Jeremy's grades went from D's and E's to A's and B's. He also began working at a restaurant nearby and began calling himself Rob instead of Jeremy.

It looked like his childhood problems were in his past and our little family of three was beginning to be happy.

We bought our very own townhouse near Lakeville, which had a Rosemount address and Apple Valley phone number, although Domino's pizza assumed we lived in Farmington. We got a pretty good deal. The townhouse was three levels and had three bedrooms, two bathrooms, a living room with fireplace, and a family room. We went out and got a cat named Jingles who fit in fairly quickly.

Within two months of ownership, just about Christmas time, I got a call from my sister to tell me my mother had lung cancer and would be having surgery on December 26. Steve and I packed up the car on the twenty-third and began the twelve-hour drive to Detroit, Michigan. I did all the driving as Steve said his stomach was feeling queasy. We stopped at several rest stops along the way while Steve was sick. I drove while he slept most of the way He was feeling better when we arrived at my Mother's apartment the next morning. It was his first time to meet his in-laws. I was unable to walk after driving such a long way, and Steve had to support me as I made my way to the door. I was shaking like a leaf and concern shifted from my mother's health to my health. My family was alarmed at the changes that I had been experiencing so gradually that I hadn't noticed. I was unable to talk and asked to be allowed to sleep immediately.

When I woke up about four hours later, I felt pretty normal again. My family was still concerned about my health and insisted that as soon as I got back to Minnesota I should see a doctor. I promised so I could get the attention off me and back on my mom. I had been to Michigan to visit my mother and sisters at least once a year since moving to Minnesota. In all the time I resided in Minnesota I had not received a visit from any of them.

My mother would call fairly regularly, but I was lucky if I received one letter a year from either of my sisters. My brave second eldest sister, had been diagnosed with multiple sclerosis when she was in her midtwenties. Even in High School, I noticed her odd posture. She walked with her hips thrown forward, ahead of her body. She achieved her lifelong dream to be a nurse. She got married after nursing school, first converting to Judaism to please her future husband and mother-in-law. She has taught around the United States at seminars for training of nurses. She also goes to Europe or another country once a year ago as a vacation and is an amateur photographer. She chose to have no children. She and her husband, a biologist, reside in an upscale suburb of Detroit called Huntington Woods.

My eldest sister had dreams in her high school days of being a wife and mom and to try work as a beautician. She went to beautician school but dropped out when little old ladies, who had their hair styled once a week, left their hair as it was styled. When they came in for their weekly or biweekly wash and style without having washed or combed their hair since their last appointment, they encouraged bugs to lodge in their hair. My sister decided that even with latex gloves to protect her from touching the bugs, she was too squeamish for the job.

She did achieve her goal to be a mom, and she was the best. Her son, Thomas, never lacked for love and affection. My sister worked in a job she still works to this day to be sure there was food on the table for her son. He went to Wayne University and received his teaching degree in math and physics. He married and moved far north to Cheboygan, Michigan, where he had been offered a job so his mother very rarely gets to see him or her new grandchild.

The year my mother was diagnosed with lung cancer, my sisters brought food and gifts on Christmas day, and we spent it together. The following day, my mother was prepared for surgery. We all stayed in the waiting room (my sisters, Steve, and I) to see what the outcome would be. My middle sister's husband is not the family sort and avoids contact with any member of the family as much as possible. The wait for the procedure seemed a long time. After the long wait, the surgeon came out in his surgical scrubs to let us know that he thought her odds of surviving the surgery were good. He believed he got it all, and they had also taken biopsies of lymph nodes in the area to test for cancer cells. He also told us lung surgery is one of the most painful of surgeries, and it would take a long time for her to recover. We snuck a peak of her in ICU and could barely see any of her as she was covered from head to toe with breathing apparatus and monitors. Since she would be anesthetized for the rest of the day, we all went to our various homes. Steve and I were staying in my mother's apartment home.

We stayed a few more days and then headed back to Minnesota so that Steve could be there for the first day of the new school year. I celebrated my thirty-fifth birthday on January 6, and true to my word, I called my internist and set up a doctor's appointment, sure that I would be told to slow down, that there was no problem other than stress.

Chapter 6

The Diagnosis, Denial, and Acceptance

I felt silly as I sat and waited in the waiting room to see the doctor. I always hated going to the doctor. When I had gone in the past, several years ago, I was having frightful headaches, and they attributed them to stress and recommended aspirin. I honestly felt I was probably doing too much as I was still six months shy of getting my bachelor's degree and working two jobs. When my name was called, I resigned myself to following through and followed the nurse to the examining room. Blood pressure as usual was quite low. I walked daily still so was in excellent physical condition. Weight, 125. Height, 5 foot 5 inches. Pulse in the 70s. And normal temperature. The nurse asked me why I was there, and I explained my family's reaction when I was in Michigan the month before and that I was fulfilling my promise to see a doctor when I got home. She told me the doctor would be there soon and left the room.

I sat there feeling more and more foolish for taking up the doctor's time. He finally knocked and entered the door. I once more explained why I had come, and he listened very patiently. My leg jiggled up and down constantly while I talked, and my fingers kept rolling as if I had a coin in my hand. When he asked me about these off movements, I responded that I had a very busy schedule, and it was just nervous reflexes. He said he thought I should be seen by a neurologist and made me an appointment to see one the next day. This made me a bit nervous, and when I went home and told Steve and Jeremy, Steve just laughed the news off and said it was probably nothing.

The next day found me sitting in a St. Paul downtown clinic in a neurology examining room alone, waiting to see the neurologist, Dr. XXX1. When he entered the examining room, he was all business. He made me imitate what appeared to me to be child games. Open your hands and shut them very fast. Touch your finger to your nose and then my finger, back to your nose, moving his finger to a different spot each time. Tap your foot on the floor as fast as you can. After several of these childish games, he checked my reflexes and manipulated my arms. After this, he opened the door of the examining room and had me walk to the end of the hall and back. Finally, he was done, and I was waiting for his diagnosis back in the examining room. "You have Parkinson's disease," he stated. He handed me a prescription for Selegine and told me to come back in six months. When he left the room, I could hardly breathe.

How could he tell from those silly tests that I had a disease? I didn't have a disease; I was just stressed out. What was Parkinson's disease? How much longer did I have to live? Would this kill me? My mind was searching to make sense of this diagnosis. At the moment, I was alone with this knowledge and had to drive myself home with my mind unable to focus on driving and trying to deal with the shock I had just received. I finally arrived home, my head spinning with the terrible news. When I walked into the house, Steve and Jeremy were laughing at a joke Jeremy heard in school that day. Steve and Jeremy could both tell something was wrong the minute they saw my face. I took all my anger and fear and directed it at them. "Did you forget I had a neurology appointment today?" I could see Steve had while Jeremy just sat silent. "I have Parkinson's disease!" I exclaimed and began to cry. Steve came over to comfort me. "What is Parkinson's disease?" he asked as he walked over toward me to hold me while I cried. "I don't know! Leave me alone!" I screamed at him, ran up the stairs into our bedroom, and slammed the door. I always denied Steve the need to comfort me without realizing how it hurt him. I wanted to be in control of my feelings. I didn't want to need anyone. Needing someone made you vulnerable. I cried myself to sleep and woke up later when the house was dark. I got up and went downstairs. Steve was still up, but Jeremy had gone to bed. I had been angry at Steve for laughing off my neurology appointment the day before. But now I was ready to grieve with him at the loss of my health. Steve is one of the most patient men in the world and allowed me into his arms for comforting. Neither of us knew what we were fighting so were more frightened than we needed to be.

Being a student at St. Catherine's with an Information Management major made me very computer literate. At the time I was diagnosed, I had an internet account when the internet was still in its infancy. Through the use of the internet, I was able to learn more and more about what Parkinson's symptoms were. In the sixteen years I have lived with the diagnosis, I still do not know what Parkinson's is and neither do the neurologists. My venturing onto the internet brought me up against my first ethical question I would need to research in order to live with my illness.

I had found a web site called the Dumpster Gang that was intended as a both a support group and self advocacy group for persons with Parkinson's disease. I introduced myself to the group and was welcomed with open arms. I read all the posts posted thus far. One post particularly bothered me. The poster insisted that all of us must unite and be self-advocates for Parkinson's disease. I was not ready to make my illness the priority in my life. I still had children to raise and a degree to attain. Since she challenged everyone on the site to express their opinion, I decided to answer her question. I politely pointed out that I had children to spend time with and a degree to attain. After that, I did not want the stress that would be brought on by advocating for a cure. I did not believe all the replies I received from my post. All were negative. I was called selfish by many. Some warned me if I didn't advocate for a cure, then no one would. Others pointed out the stress in their lives but their devotion to advocate for Parkinson's disease took first priority. They complained how unfair it was that I might benefit from their advocating. I once more tried to explain that though I admired them for their advocating efforts,

I had had too much stress in my life and felt I had earned the right to live my way by putting my family first and integrating my disease into the mix. At this point, the husband of the first poster who issued the challenge for all persons with Parkinson's to advocate accused me of personally trying to hurt his wife's feelings by answering her challenge with a negative reply and used some colorful language to make a direct attack upon me. He defended his wife by telling some of the bad things that had happened to her. I became very angry at his interference and explained my childhood and the abuse I had undergone, so I felt I had the right to live what was left of my life as I saw fit. At this point, I stopped reading and posting on this site for a long time.

What does it mean to be a "self advocate" when you are the patient with the illness? Should you direct, through grant money raised, who and what should be researched about your disease? Can you claim you are the only one who understands what your disease and others with the same diagnosis feel like living with it? Or should you try to educate your doctor, neurologist, and movement disorder specialist? I hope, through describing my experiences living with this disease, to address the above issues.

Chapter 7

And the Diagnosis Is Definitely, Well Maybe, Could Be . . .

About the time I was diagnosed, stem cells were just beginning to become an issue in the Parkinson community. One of the members of a support group I had joined had in fact allowed himself to be in a study where he had embryonic stem cells implanted in his brain. I observed no improvement in his condition, and he died of heart failure a short while later. My husband and I continued to attend support group meetings, but everyone was so much older than I, and the group leaders directed the meeting so as not to allow patients to get off topic, so we both lost interest in attending. I continued on with my life, continuing to educate myself about the illness and losing my anger and denial and moved into acceptance. I went through depression, milder than my past depression, but realizing it was a secondary symptom of Parkinson's, I went to a psychiatrist and worked on dealing with it. Steve was so wonderful to me that I found all my distrust of him evaporating, and our fighting, usually ending up with my threatening to leave him, stopped. I trusted him every day. I also made the decision to choose my battles and not fight over every little thing. I did a lot of growing that year, thanks to Steve's example.

Jeremy was doing very well in school and was chosen to do a business internship during his senior year and write a paper about it. He also finally earned enough money to buy his own car, which he was very proud of. He enlisted in the army during his senior year. What seemed a good idea at the time ended up to be a mistake. He graduated and went for basic training. I expect the constant in-your-face method of training was too much like the bullying he took as a child in elementary school. Fortunately he and the army found out he was not a good military candidate, and they medically discharged him. He came back to Steve, and I deeply changed. He no longer wanted to work or consider school. I believe he thought himself a failure in everyone's eyes. He only wanted to be left alone to play video games. Both Steve and I insisted he find work. Now, looking back, I think psychological counseling would have been the better choice. He bought a mobile home and found a job and a roommate. Unfortunately, Jeremy made poor choices in friends, and his roommates didn't work, pay their half of the rent, and turned his mobile home into a dump.

Jeremy delivered pizza's until his car gave out. He sold the mobile home to one of his roommates' friends and moved in with his dad.

Joseph did not follow up to make sure Jeremy told him the truth. Jeremy, not wanting to disappoint his Dad, would lie and say he found a job at a local restaurant; his dad believed him, and Jeremy stayed home and played video games once more. I continued to see James and Jared. After years of participation in the Boy Scouts, both of them were promoted to Eagle Scout. If it was not for their father's support and encouragement, they would not have achieved the highest rank in scouting. I attended all the football games they marched in the band for, all their concerts, and was surprised when James decided to join the army reserves.

One night about 10:30 PM, I received a call from James. James always was the one who took care of things now. He was fighting back tears as he told me their seventeen-year-old cat, Sasha, was on the couch crying in pain. She had been there most of the evening, but the boys could not convince Joseph to take her to the vet. Was there anything I could do to help her?

I jumped out of bed, dressed, and rushed over to the boys' house. It was exactly as James described. Poor Sasha was lying on the couch in extreme pain. I told both of the boys, James and Jared, that I would take her to an emergency veterinary clinic I knew of, but considering her age and the extent of pain she was in, the kindest thing would probably be was to have her put down. Both of the boys were old enough to understand what I was telling them and agreed with me. They gave her a last hug and kiss, and then I took her to the vet and stayed while she was euthanized. It was done very gently and with dignity. I had tears streaming down my face as I paid the fee and left the clinic. I called the children to let them know what had happened, and they took the news stoically.

By this time, Jared was fed up with his Dad's ignoring Jeremy's behavior. It seemed that he had begun choosing worse friends to hang out with that were teaching him easy ways to make money and buy drugs. Jared called me in his senior year of high school to tell me Jeremy had friends in when his father was not home and they were doing drugs. If the drugs were discovered, James could be court-martialed for living in the same house. This time both Steve and I went over. Jeremy was not home at the time, and I called the police. They arrived and searched his room with my permission. They found drugs, and when Jeremy came home, he was arrested for possession.

Frustrated by Jeremy's behavior, Jared asked to live with Steve and I, and we said no problem. James chose to stay at his Dad's house. When Joseph got home later that evening, the police told him they had found drugs, had arrested Jeremy and advised Joseph that he should not allow Jeremy to continue living in his house. Joseph claimed Jeremy was working as a busboy at a local restaurant as far as he knew and had been for two years. When Steve and I called the restaurant, they had never even heard of Jeremy. It was a very long time before I heard from Jeremy again. He would call his Dad whenever he needed cash because he knew his Dad felt guilty and would provide him with it. Soon afterward, Jeremy began driving a cab, seemed to enjoy the line of work, and was well suited for it. We once more were communicating.

Meanwhile, my Parkinson's was gradually making itself known. I had been on Sinemet 25/100 for about two years now and was seeing a new neurologist.

Her neurology consult notes for April 2, 1996 read as follows:

This is a follow-up for a 42 year old woman with Parkinson's disease. The patient has increased her Sinemet to four times a day occasionally, and is tolerating the selegiline twice a day, with overall beneficial results. The patient notes less rigidity. She also brings in an article commenting about increased mortality in patients taking selegiline.

She has not needed to use the Lososyn for side effects from the Sinemet thus far. The patient's foremost problem today is insomnia. Since last seen, approximately 3 months ago, the patient believes she has had 3 nights of uninterrupted sleep. Last evening, for example, the patient went to sleep at 10:30, awakened at 11:30, and essentially was unable to sleep all night. She did try Restoril which was beneficial 2-3 nights, and subsequently was no longer effective. The patient indicates that she can take the Restoril, use a wine cooler and still is unable to fall asleep.

Review of the chart indicates the patient tried Permax in the past, which caused dizziness and vomiting.

The patient feels that she is not depressed at this time, but primarily sleep deprived and although does have a history of depression, using medications, she does not feel hopeless at this time, and feels involved with life.

Medications: Sinemet 25/100 t.i.d. or q.i.d., selegiline 5 mg. p.o. b.i.d., Restoril 15 mg q.h.s.

Blood Pressure 106/78, heart rate 60. Mental status: The patient is alert. She is somewhat depressed about her problem with insomnia. There is no voice tremor. Cranial nerves notable for masking of facies. Motor exam: There is some paratonia in the upper extremities. Gait: The patient has fairly fluid gait with decreased associated arm swing in her right arm, but does have associated arm swing in the left arm.

Parkinson's with significant insomnia. In my opinion, treatment of the insomnia would be beneficial for this patient's overall disease. We will give her a trial of Clonopin which will help some of the restless legs as well as help her with sleep. If she does develop tolerance to this, then we will try her on Ambien. We will also arrange for the patient to be studied at the Hennepin County Sleep Laboratory for any further recommendations beyond that. We will not refer the patient to Health Psychology

at this time, until the sleep disorder is further managed.
The patient will return in six weeks time.

Visit Diagnosis: Sleep Stage Dysfunctions and Paralysis
agitans

By this time, I was on disability. I worked for two years for a law firm as the assistant to the Information Manager until I could no longer lift the heavy boxes of paper bills onto the shelves. I began working part-time for a veterinarian office cleaning up after dogs and cats and shampooing some of the dogs. I could not pick up the heavier breeds after a while so left that position. I applied for social security at my doctor's urging and was accepted the first try.

In June of 1996, I was seen for a neurology consultation by a psychologist. His entry in my medical chart reads as follows:

Presenting Problem
Dianna Lynn is a 42 year old married female diagnosed
with Parkinson's disease since 1991. She is seen by me at the
request of her treating neurologist regarding evaluation
of the psycho/social problems that she has current and in
her past and the relationship of those psycho/social issues
to management of her Parkinson condition.

Background Information:

Dianna is 42 years of age, currently unemployed, but employed in the past as a musician. Her husband age 45 is a musician and teacher.

Dianna is unemployed at this point due to the debilitating/ disabling effects of her Parkinson's condition.

This is a second marriage for both of them. They have children from previous relationships. Dianna's first marriage was entered into primarily as a way to get away from her home situation which included sexual abuse at the hands of her father.

Dianna indicates that between the ages of 13 and 18 there was regular sexual abuse occurring.

As she began to resist father's advances more regularly he would fill a bag with propane gas and essentially asphyxiate Dianna to the point that she would become more submissive to his advances.

Dianna indicates that she has gone through months of psychotherapy designed to help her resolve problems stemming from this abuse. This psychotherapy has also included involvement in group therapy approaches. She indicates that the result of all that treatment was quite positive. She went back to school to take control of her life. Ironically and tragically at the point that she was ready to graduate, she began to exhibit the Parkinson's symptoms. For Dianna, the onset of the Parkinson's has reactivated issues related to the abuse in that she once again feels there is something happening to her over which she has little control.

From this point on I will continue to share my medical records, leaving out the patient history to reduce repetition in this book.

Transcription

Neurology Consult

Author: Dr. XXX (new neurologist as former moved from state)

History: I was asked to evaluate this 44-year old female with the diagnosis of Parkinson's disease. She was previously followed by Dr. YYY.

Apparently Ms. Lynn has a history of Parkinson's disease diagnosed about 10 years earlier. The details are really unknown to me at this time. She has had a number of different medications for this and currently is taking Sinemet, Eldepryl and Mirapex. She notes that since the Artane was discontinued back in December of 1997 when she last saw Dr. YYY and after Mirapex was started that she has less difficulty with wearing off. She had some nausea initially but this passed.

She indicates that her Parkinson's symptoms are exaggerated with her menstrual period. She uses Premarin 0.625 mg. 5 days prior to her period. What benefit this gives her I don't know. She also indicates her Parkinson's disease is increased with stress. She has had no significant change in her condition over the last six to nine months.

Social History: In spite of her Parkinson's disease, she remains an active individual. She is a musician and plays in a salsa band (actually I played in a Sousa Band). *She also plays for a number of theatrical productions for several local theatres. Her Parkinson's disorder does not prevent her from doing these activities.*

Medications: Current medications are Mirapex (0.25 mg.) 2 tablets two to three times a day, Sinemet CR (50/100) 1 tav QHS. Sinemet CR (25/100) 1 tab two times per day (9:00am - 4:00pm.) Eldepryl (5 mg.) 1 tab two times per day (9:00 am and 4:00 pm.) Premarin (0.625 mg.) five days prior to her menstrual period.

Physical Examination: On examination, blood pressure 110/70. Pulse 80. Mental status: She was alert and oriented X 3. Speech was normal. Recent and remote memory and concentration were normal. She avoided eye contact and tended to hold her head and look toward the floor and the left. Cranial nerves: Visual fields full to confrontation. Pupils, equal, round and reactive to light. EOM's intact. Fundiscopic examination appeared benign bilaterally. Face was symmetric there appeared to be good facial power and good bilaterally. The tongue and uvula were midline. There were no fascicualations or tremors or abnormal movements of the tongue. Sensation normal to light touch and double simultaneous stimulation over all four extremeties and both sides of the face.

Motor: Normal bulk, tone and strength in all muscle groups. I really did not appreciate any increased tone. There was no cogwheeling on today's examination. She had very bizarre tremors. These were not the classic pill-rolling or rhymic tremor that one typically sees in Parkinson's disease.

She had shaking of her legs which was basically bouncing off her legs up and down on the floor. This was bilateral, it was varied in amplitude and was alternating with one leg going up and the other was going down. She also had this type of a tremor in her hands where her hands were bouncing around on her leg. She had tremor of her head which involved the side to side or "no-no" tremor as well. The tremors would come and go throughout the examination. Reflexes sere 2+ and symmetric and toes sere down going bilaterally Coordination of finger-nose-finger and rapid alternating movements were symmetric in the upper extremities. She had the most bizarre gait that I had seen in a long while. This was somewhat antalgic in appearance. She tended to walk with a somewhat stooped posture and tended to list to the left as she walked in the hall. She could walk on heels and toes without much difficulty. She could perform a tandem without using the wall for support.

Assessment: History of Parkinson's disease. This I have to admit is the most bizarre presentation of Parkinson's disease I have seen. I am not at all convinced that it is true Parkinson's disease.

The details and the description of the events at the onset are unclear to me at this time. It is clear however that she has firmly implanted this idea that this is Parkinson's and this is shared by her husband. In spite of the wild tremor, she is active. She does not have any other associated symptoms of Parkinson's. In fact I could not appreciate any true mask facies. She has no brandykinesia and no increased tone. She has no associated symptoms such as drooling or constipation.

Clearly, there are a number of psychological issues that she has not completely dealt with. She was in counseling for a while and Dr. MMM actually saw her. Alter for a number of visits However, she discontinued that therapy with the excuse being that transportation was difficult. I am not sure what to make out of her history of the asphyxiation with propane. Propane is not a typical gas that he would use for welding. It is unclear to me what would also happen or potentially happen while she was unconscious.

Plan: At this time, since the diagnosis remains unclear to me, I decided not to make any changes in her medications. In spite of this diagnosis of Parkinson's disease and her wild tremor, she remains really quite active. I will take this opportunity to review her chart and try to determine whether her initial presentation really supports the diagnosis of Parkinson's disorder. I also suggested that they reconsider psychological counseling. There does appear to be some difficulties with regard to the marriage, and I think this could only be of benefit to the two of them. However, at this time, I don't have a good feeling that she is inclined to pursue that. I asked them to return in 6 months for further evaluation

Visit diagnosis: **Multiple Sclerosis and Depressive Disorder**

[Multiple Sclerosis? I believe when I was originally diagnosed, an MRI was ordered, which showed no scarred tissue of my brain, which ruled out this disorder.]

Neurology Consult: 10-24-2000

Subjective: This is a follow-up visit for this 46 year old female with a diagnosis of Parkinson's disease. Dianna comes today accompanied by her husband. She brings in a two page typed list of problems. The first thing she notes is that she increased her Mirapex for the total dose of 6 mg per day as directed at the time of her last visit. Disturbance and sudden crying without apparent reason, feelings of hopelessness, etc. occurred when she took the higher dosage. There was no major change in her life or significant stress at the time. She changed her dose back down to the previous level still has some difficulty with a sleep disturbance.

She notes she has trouble with the effect of Sinemet and Mirapex at the time of her period. Apparently five days before she seems to have some Provera during this time which seems to help. Once the period comes she has rapid improvement of effect if the Sinemet and Mirapex. She also notes that that she has been giving more difficulty with ridgidity on the right side of her body. This has caused more difficulty with balance and she had some dyskinesias of the foot. She feels more clumsy with the right upper extremity as well. She driving is much more difficult because of the difficulty with the right extremity.

She notes that late in the day she may have some wearing off symptoms. She has more difficulty towards the end of the day. She also notes that she is having more difficulty with cognitive processes and two and three part tasks are difficult for her to complete.

Medications:
Medications are taken at 5:00 AM, 11:00 AM, 5:00 PM and 10:00 PM.
Sinemet (25.100) 1-0-0-0
Sinemet CR (25/100) 0-1-1-1
Mirapex 1 mg (1-1-1-1)
Eldepryl (5 mg) 0-1-1-0
Provera ((10mg) 1 tablet at onset of period.

Physical Examination: On examination, blood pressure 100/74, pulse 96m weight 155lb., height 165', General examination revealed a well developed female in no acute distress. Extracular movements intact. Cranial nerves were normal. She has some paucity of facial movement. She had good strength throughout all extremities. She does have brandykinesia and some increase in tone, a little bit more notable on the right side than the left but this is really very mild and minimal at today's examination. She had no dysmetria with finger-nose-finger. She did have intermittent tremor in the extremities, most notable in the lower extremities on today's visit. Her casual gait was abnormal and somewhat saddling. She had a slightly increased base, shortened stride length. She used a cane for balance assistance again on her right, and as she was plodding down the hall in a somewhat forced propulsive manner, she ran into the view box and a chart holder that suspended down the hall. Romberg was absent. I did not attempt to have her perform a tandem.

Assessment: Ms. Lynn carries a diagnosis of Parkinson's disease based on early assessments. She has a very odd gait and in comparison with what had seen six months ago, her gait is entirely different. The shaking and "tremor" of her limbs is fairly similar to what I saw before and that is much harder to describe and correlate from time to time. I really do question the diagnosis of Parkinson's disease because this looks just so very odd.

However, she has been given this diagnosis and now both she and her husband are convinced that this is what she has and want to continue working with the medication because they believe it is having some effect. [If you don't believe me, how can you help me?] *Therefore, we will continue to pursue that while we collect a little more information and get some time to see her on multiple occasions At this point, we will continue to increase the Mirapex since I think it is relatively benign. It supposedly gave her some improvement in* *her symptoms and therefore we will try to see what we can get out of this medication. She will increase her total Mirapex dose by two tablets by adding one half tablet per day over the course of the next four weeks. At that time, I would like to have her return for another visit and further observation.*

Plan:

1. *Continue Sinemet immediately release and Sinemet CR as well as eldepryl at the current doses and the current times. She was instructed to make no change in these doses or rimes without consulting me.*

2. *Increase Mirapex by adding ½ tablet (0.5 mg) every week for the next four weeks. At the end of her titration, she will be taking one half tablet at 0530 and one and a half tablets at 1000 and the 1700 and 2300. A detailed titration schedule was provided in writing.*

3. *Detailed counseling was provided. She was asked to call if she had any adverse effect from the additions. She was also asked to call at the end of five weeks to report her status.*

4. *RTC 2 months, sooner P.R.N*

Diagnosis: Abnormality of Gait

Chapter 8

Cascading Effects from Loss of Dopamine

Had the doctor asked me as to why my legs were shaking in such an odd way, I would have told him the symptoms he was observing at that particular moment in time were caused by restless legs syndrome and were not my Parkinson's symptoms. Now this was a young neurologist who was accustomed to seeing children, not adults. He did not specialize in movement disorders. I always hated when I would tell my neurologist that I was having a problem and they would explain that the problem had nothing to do with Parkinson's disease. The neurologist I was seeing refused to admit it was possible my menses could be affected by my Parkinson's disease. His conclusion was based on a compilation of interviews of younger women with Parkinson's (a sampling of fifty), which came to the conclusion that a woman's period was unaffected by Parkinson's (see exhibit C). I actually sent an e-mail to the author of the survey and asked why she had not taken a more scientific study, for example, the measurement of specific hormones. She responded that the grant being offered specifically spelled out the study must be a survey. The Movement Disorder Experts and the Neurological Fields were not looking at the different studies being done outside their field of study to discover what are called the cascading effects of Parkinson's disease.

Gynecological Cascading Symptoms

Women Parkinson patients have been speculating about the effect of the menstrual cycle on their Parkinson's symptoms for years. The week before the period, the effectiveness of the patients' drugs ability to work is vastly affected. There are numerous studies that show the role of dopamine in the reproductive system:

> Time-dependent effects of oestradiol and progesterone on hypothalamic catecholamine turnover in ovariectomized rats. Results showed the increase of noradrenaline turnover in the POAG was accompanied by a low afternoon turnover rate of dopamine in the MBH. The results support that the view that the induction of LH afternoon surges depends upon an increase of stimulatory noradrenergic inputs to the POAH and a decrease of inhibitory dopaminergic inputs in the MBH.[1]

The mechanism through which oestrogen influences striatal function to affect behavior in the female is sexually dimorphic (in English, has two effects.) Experiments In my laboratory have shown that oestrogen influences the activity of striatal dopamine terminals and has effects on striatal dopamine receptors. We have also shown that there are sex differences in the basal extracellular concentration of dopamine in the striatum, and in the rapid effect of a single injection of oestrogen on the behavioral and neurochemical responses to drugs such amphetamine that induce dopamine release. Furthermore there are sex differences in the rapid and acute effects of oestrogen on striatal dopamine receptor binding that mirror the hormonal effects on striatal dopamine release.[2]

Abnormal regulation of prolactin release in idiopathic Parkinson's disease.[3]

The truth is dopamine plays a major role in the woman's ability to breast-feed her child as dopamine is the primary neuron released by the brain to regulate how much prolactin is released into a woman's body. Yet the only study doctors will give credence to is a survey taken by Parkinson's women in childbearing years that stated they had no worsening of their symptoms when they experienced menses, which was done by a Movement Disorder Clinic, not a gynecological group. If you suspect your menses are affected by the levodopa/carbadopa, do not speak to your neurologist. Speak to your gynecologist.

Cascading Psychological Symptoms

The brain is more complicated than any other part of the body. Millions of different chemicals act as a check and balance system in the brain. Too little dopamine has cascading effects since it acts as a check on how much serotonin is released in the system. Serotonin is known as causing pleasure. No pleasurable sensation leads to depression and anxiety. Patients are aware of this and have known this for years. Yet neurologists do not listen to the patients when they tell them this; they wait until someone has done a study of rat brains or some other model, then read the study, and believe it because of the scientific methodology of the test. Read the following discussion of a Parkinson's forum on exactly this topic:

First poster: PD and anxiety disorders?

The further down the PD road I get the more I wonder about its link with anxiety disorders. It's occurred to me more than once that we are a group of people who are either shaking or frozen stiff—both manifestations of fear [a.k.a anxiety]. I have tried to sidestep the whole business of anxiety with an "I've got a grip on life" attitude, but lately that has been crumbling and I do believe that I have, among my collection of lives' trinkets, an anxiety disorder. As a matter of fact I'm wondering if the whole PD package is rooted in anxiety [As a man thinketh ...] *You could say I've reached the point where:*

1. *I admit that I am powerless over anxiety, and that my life has become unmanageable.*
   a. *Have come to believe that a Power greater than myself (possibly [more] drugs?) can restore me to sanity.*
2. *Have made a decision to turn my life over to a good psychotherapist.*
3. *Made a searching and fearless [???] mental inventory of myself.*
   a. *Have admitted to God, myself and my doctors the exact nature of my anxieties ... etc. [Should I continue to 12?] What are your thoughts on anxiety and PD, I know I'm not alone.*

The wisdom of this poster is evident. Her/his decision to go to a psychologist is right on. Just as Dr. Patterson from the APDA said that all emergency staff cannot be expected to know everything, the treating neurologist is exactly the same, even more so. The neurologist has a tough job. He/she is working in a field that is only in its infancy. With the Genome project, we are learning just how complicated the brain is and how it interacts through the nervous system, endocrine system, and other body systems to keep everything in the body working well together. Therefore, if you find your symptom is what could be called a cascading symptom (a symptom that occurs because of the lack of dopamine), then you should be going to the type of doctor who specializes in that capacity.

But that is the irony of Parkinson's. It is a life filled with lucidness or confusion. The people who are caretakers of the Parkinson's patient are expected to know which mood the patient is in. When they cannot tell and treat the patient as being confused when the patient is lucid, trust fails in the relationship.

Cascading Optical Symptoms

I have been having difficulties with my eye and eye movements. When I am in a car, I constantly feel as if it is about to be hit by the cars on either side. A large truck passing on the right or left of the car I am riding in always seems to be pulling toward the car I am riding in. I brought this up to my neurologist who said he had never heard of Parkinson's affecting the eyes. He/she only reads his specialty newsletters put out by the Neurological Institute he/she is a member of. They do not have time to read Ophthalmology Medical Journals on the offhand chance that it might have an article that may affect their specialty.

I asked my treating neurologist if he knew any effect Parkinsonism would have on the eyes. I was fifty years old and already was showing signs of a detached retina and had cataracts in both of my eyes. His response was he had never heard of anything.

I did some of my own research on the internet and found the following:

Mechanisms of the Basal Ganglia: Role of Dopamine

Dopamine (DA) is a critical determinant of basal ganglia function. DA neurons located in the substantia nigra pars compacta (SNc) and its vicinity project to the striatum (in addition to frontal cortical and limbic areas) and exert strong modulatory influences over the corticostriatal signal transmission. Patients with Parkinson's disease, which is caused by the degenerations of DA neurons show deficits in eye movements.[4]

A large amount of information is processed in the brain simultaneously, but an optimal behavior under a particular behavioral context requires the selection of information that is appropriate for the particular context. Attention, in its broadest sense, indicates such a selection process.[5]

The same article also explains why a Parkinson's patient may have problems with working memory, relation to expectation (a mental state evoked by a predictive event) as well as the relation to sequential procedural learning causing difficulties.

Notes

1. Journal of Endocrinology, Vol. 106, Issue 3 (1985), 303-309.
2. Becker, J. B., Dept. of Psychology, Reproductive Sciences Program, University of Michigan, Ann Arbor, USA.
3. *Journal of Psycho Pharmacy*, Vol. 17, pp. 2004-2009.
4. *Psychological Review*, Vol. 80, No. 3, July 2000, pp. 954-970.
5. *Psychological Review*, Vol. 80, No. 3, July 2000, pp. 954-970.

Chapter 9

Meanwhile, In My Ordinary Life

The last chapter was so full of medical transcriptions, I am afraid you may have forgotten I am also a living person outside of the Parkinson's disease. While all the medical visits were happening, my life did not stop. I was encouraged by a close and dear friend who managed the schools for a local music store to consider giving private studio lessons at her store to students beginning music lessons for the first time. I was very flattered to be thought of as a person able to teach. I took her up on her offer and began teaching students for the store.

About the same time, my husband decided he would like to go for his Master's Degree in order to increase his salary to a higher lane path. He was informed of the perfect Master's Program for working band teachers by a friend who was already attending the program.

It only took three years to complete, and all work was done in the summer during an intense three week period. The cost was high but affordable. The program was in Southern Oregon, and it would mean leaving me to my own resources with the inability to drive. It seemed to be so important to Steve to have his Master's Degree, so I agreed with him that he should go. I insisted he take only three years to finish and that he had to commit once he started. He was in total agreement. He left for Portland the next summer for his first year. The program was refined for band directors. The program had a set curriculum that included each of the instrument families (Brass, Percussion, and Woodwind) with each instrument being addressed for educational purposes by a professional instrumentalist, usually with a doctorate degree for the instrument of study. Each candidate was also given an opportunity to direct a piece and his performance of the piece was taped and critiqued by a professional conductor. Music theory was covered technologically by introduction of computer programs to run classrooms or for composition purposes. Each student was also expected to choose a project to work on during the summer.

Meanwhile back home, I was working on a project that would take the entire three weeks he was gone to complete. I ripped out the downstairs carpeting and sanded and stained the hardwood floors beneath.

Steve was very enthusiastic about his experience over the past three weeks when he arrived at home. He was also amazed at the change in our townhouse. The next year flew by as I continued to teach in the music studio and helped Steve with his inner-city schools, and soon summer was approaching. Steve barely had enough money saved up for tuition and the airfare to go back the second year. He also had not completed his summer project. If he left me at home by myself, I would have less than $50 to see me through until he returned. Steve was embarrassed to have to admit to the director that he had not done his project. He tried to convince me he shouldn't go because we were so low on money. I firmly told him we had both committed to his continuing his three years consecutively and told him to go. He left me at home and went back a little reluctantly this time. In a couple of days, I got a call. He had managed to talk the director into letting him finish his project before the three weeks were over for that year and, from then on, enjoyed the classes and applied himself harder.

This time when he was gone, I tackled the second largest bedroom upstairs. With the experience of the prior year, I had learned a lot and did a much better job. Once more, after his three weeks of school, Steve came home happy as a clam and was very complementary on my home improvement efforts. He had more confidence and was excited to realize he had only one more year and he would have his Master's Degree. His father was quite proud of him. The next school year passed much as the one before. My Parkinson's was gradually worsening, but I felt confident I would be OK for the three weeks it would take him the next summer to complete his degree.

When Steve came back, he seemed changed somehow. He seemed to resent my being in his classrooms that year, so I stopped coming. He stopped asking my opinion on problems he had with the classes like he used to. He began spending more and more time at school rather than coming home. When he did come home, he went straight to bed. When it was time to go for his last year, he was anxious to go, and to be perfectly honest, I was ready for him to go as a quiet tension had grown between the two of us and I needed and wanted some space from him.

Once more, Steve left for college. This time I was unable to complete more than take the carpet off the Master Bedroom floor. When he called, he could hear the tired sound in my voice and was very concerned. When he came home for the final time, we both were euphoric and relieved. Steve was proud of his accomplishment. His senior class project was published in the Band Director's Digest. But I sensed a change in his emotions and attitude toward me. He was pulling away. He did not need my help in his class, so I began to stay home more and more. The solitude made me focus too much on myself and my Parkinson's problems, and I failed to see how hard Steve was working to keep us financially afloat. He worked all day and had to rush home to get me to the studio in time for my first lesson. Since I taught three days a week and was now averaging forty-five students, he was stuck in the parking lot or at the McDonald's next door, waiting for me to finish. He spent the time working on keeping his classroom records up. I never thanked him for his hard schedule to enable me to continue teaching. Steve was also beginning to put on weight as he ate fast food almost every day. He was also beginning to feel the letdown that comes when you have completed a goal successfully as he had done and have nothing to work toward that would bring him the same recognition. I began giving up students and cutting back on my teaching schedule, which only made me harder to live with because I was alone more and more.

On the nights I gave up teaching, Steve would stay after school and have fast food dinners. By the time he got home, he was so tired that he would only want to sleep.

I finally cut out teaching altogether and did only occasional shows to give him more time. But he still kept finding reasons to work later and still was too tired to talk when he came home. It was no small wonder that he wanted to avoid me because my favorite topic of conversation was my Parkinson's disease. He had been hearing of little else, and between exhaustion and my nagging, he finally broke down one day and said he wanted a divorce. I had put complete faith in our commitment to our marriage and had stopped threatening to leave years ago when I saw the pain I put him through. I could see he was suffering now.

Steve began to lose his temper more and more frequently. He even forced me out of the car at a gas station, drove off, and left me there. I used my cell phone to get a ride home. Sometimes when we were in the car and he was frustrated by a conversation, he would use the car like a weapon, speeding and cutting back and forth across traffic, knowing that it terrified me.

This wasn't the Steve I knew. I called his best friend and asked him to try to have a talk with him and help him. I also called his younger brother Mark to see if he could help him. I pleaded with him when he said he was going to divorce me and managed somehow to get him to back down. Finally one night, he made the threat again. I began to look for spiritual help. I began reading the Bible and took a class at a local synagogue. I also went to a weekly Koran class discussion. When I reached the Prophet Jeremiah and read when he talked about how the people of Israel did not listen to God or keep his commandments and then God made a new covenant with all mankind that he would put the knowledge of God into peoples' hearts, I found him again.

Steve and I had really gotten close because we both thought that we were agnostics at the time we married. But now I knew Jesus had to exist because he had always been with me. I began to study the Bible more and more. I started from the Old Testament. I came to understand that neither I nor anyone could ever obey the commandments completely. This was why I could not fix my marriage. Also the more I learned how the brain worked, how all the different chemicals could affect each other with even the slightest change in the status quo, I knew there was no way it could happen by accident. I began to attend a Lutheran church near home. Steve was extremely surprised and suspicious. He thought I was clutching at straws by attending church. I continued to study the Bible and immerse myself in work for the church I had joined. I played my clarinet for traditional services, I substituted for the bell choir, I organized the library, but something about the church did not ring true. I hadn't joined it to find a way to make myself useful or be part of a social club. Soon the church group started what they called integrated services. I went online to discover what was the explanation for the negative changes I saw happening within the church. They began by having the music the primary emphasis for spreading God's word. I no longer volunteered my services on clarinet. I no longer felt connected to the church and called the pastor to discuss how I felt about the changes in the services. I asked him why he was giving up his honor as God's spokesman and trying to pretend that the music services were passing along the gospel and law. He accused me of not giving others the chance to share their talents. When I stated that I went to church to hear God's word and his forgiveness for my confession of my sins, he gave up and released me from membership in the church.

I joined a new church that was more traditionally oriented and felt much less uneasy with the service. This put another wedge between Steve and me. I was afraid we would never be able to repair the rift between us. The next time Steve asked me for a divorce, I left the house and took a long walk, intending never to go back. I came to realize when I got to Farmington that my motive in running away was selfish. My happiness didn't matter anymore. If Steve could not love me or commit to our marriage, my wishing he could wouldn't make it so. I felt he had done his best to make it work, and if he wasn't happy, then it was time I put my need of him aside and let him go. I walked back home and went upstairs to our bedroom and told him I would grant the divorce and not fight him over it. I told him I couldn't stand to see him in so such pain anymore and that he should move into his father's house. I came and cuddled him because he was crying. To my surprise, he told me he no longer felt he wanted a divorce but felt he should get some help. He did seek help and continues to receive mental health services. Even so, he sometimes loses his temper with me. Understandably, after all, I do have an illness that affects both my emotions and comprehension. I freely admit this. Hey, life isn't fair. Steve didn't expect to have to work so hard when we were married. I didn't realize how little time

I was going to have to feel like I was just another free person. Now that I have found true freedom through Jesus Christ, I no longer feel anger at life. It is what it is.

With my newfound faith, thanks to the Holy Spirit, I was now prepared to begin the hardest ethical argument to save my life.

Chapter 10

The Ethical Relationship between the Patient and Insurance Provider

Neurology consult

Subjective:

This is a followup visit for this 48-year-old female with Parkinson's disease. Dianna returns today accompanied by her husband. It has been some time since Dianna was in. Since her last visit in November of 2001, she has had progression of her symptoms. It is clear from today's visit that her voice is softer and she notes that people are now asking her to repeat and complaining that she is mumbling and it is difficult for them to understand her. She notes that she has had some increased difficulty swallowing.

She may choke a lot during meals. This is particularly a problem with small foods such as peas or liquids. Steak and other semi-solid foods go down much better. She has had more difficulty with balance. She rates it as "pretty bad." She fell on one occasion, spraining her ankles. She does note that she has been falling a bit more, but cannot say that she is falling in any particular direction. No significant change in bowel and bladder function. She is not constipated, but does have some stress incontinence. She blames this on a "tipped uterus." She notes that she has more cramping in the feet and legs lately than she has had in the past. With regards to the tremor, she notes that the medications are wearing off much faster than they had in the past and she is having much more fluctuation in motor control. She does get benefit out of the Sinemet and when it is functioning she is fairly well controlled and the tremor is significantly dampened. It is significantly improved so that she can continue teaching music and performing in the orchestra. She believes her on time is a couple of hours in duration. It may suddenly wear off or decrease somewhat slowly. This is really quite variable and unpredictable for her. She has a definite off period between 3 and 6 am. She tends not to use medications at this time, although she is often awake at night at about this point. At the current doses of medications she really does not have any complaints of dyskinesias.

There were no complaints of headaches, visual obscurations or loss, numbness, paresthesias or focal weakness. No chest pain, shortness of breath, abdominal. All other systems negative. Dianna today is wonder if a PET scan may be helpful for her. She has done some research on this and would like to have the test if it would be at all helpful in confirming her diagnosis and leading to improved treatment strategies. She is concerned she may have some other disorder that has been diagnosed as Parkinson's disease incorrectly.

Current Medications:

☐ *Sinemet (25/100) 1 tab 4 times a day*

☐ *Sinemet(25/1000 cr 1 Tab 4 times a day*

☐ *Mirapex (0.5 mg) 1 tab 4 times a day*

☐ *Aleve PRN*

Medication Allergies: None known

Objective:

Blood pressure 120/90, pulse: 76 weight 188 pounds. Height 65 inches. General examination revealed a well-developed female in no acute distress. Mental status was normal. She was alert and oriented x 3. She was in a good mood. Cranial nerves were intact in detail. She had good vertical gaze. There was masked facies. Her voice was hypophonic and often it was difficult to understand her. She was able to increase the amplitude of her voice when she would pay attention to the problem. Sensory examination revealed normal light touch throughout all extremities. She had good motor strength in all muscle groups. There was no dysnetria or drift of the upper extremities. She had a notable tremor that was most prominent at today's visit in the left leg and left arm. Right side has only intermittent mild tremors. This tremor was quite pronounced at the onset of the visit, but by the end of the visit, about 40 minutes later the tremor had improved significantly and she was able to sit quietly in the chair. She had taken her medications approximately a half an hour before the visit began. Casual gait was fairly normal, although her stride length was a little bit shortened. She was not able to perform a tandem.

Assessment:

Parkinsonism. We can at least say that much and she has numerous evaluations by several different individuals all confirming this is the most likely diagnosis at this point. I would agree that given her constellation of symptoms this is the most likely of the movement disorders. It is a little atypical in that she is relatively young and the tremor is quite significant. However, she does respond to the Sinemet, although at this time she is having more difficulty with the medication wearing off before the next dose. She has found the Mirapex helpful in that it helps reduce this wearing off phenomenon, but it does not eliminate it completely.

Dianna would like to participate in a study that is being conducted by the University of SSS at the V.A. Medical Center. This is involving a new agent for Parkinson's disease given via patch. To qualify for the study, however, she must discontinue the Mirapex. She requests that we make that change so that she can participate in the study. We also talked about the neurostimulator. Dianna may be a candidate for this given the fact that she is Dopamine responsive and she has significant fluctuations in motor response. However, I do not have enough expertise to make a final judgment as to whether she would or would not be a candidate in this case and so if she wants to pursue this at some point in the future, I would recommend she be seen by Dr. SSS at the University of SSS. for consideration.

I think we can make a case for a PET scan at this point. Certainly this technology has advanced significantly over the last few years and is now being shown to be helpful with the diagnoses of movement disorders. If anything it would help clarify whether this was a more typical Parkinson's disease as opposed to another of the movement disorders such as Huntington's.

Plan:

1. *Continue Sinemet (25/100) and Sinemet CR (25/100); Will increase her dose by shortening the dose interval to 1 tab every 3–4 hours as needed. She can irritate the medication based on her response. I think the shorter interval is going to be necessary as we begin tapering the Mirapex.*

2. *Taper Mirapex (0.5) mg to 0.5 tablets 4 times a day. She will do this for one week and unless there are significant adverse changes in her control, she will then drop to essentially ¼ tablet (0.125mg tabs), At that point she will change to the lower dose size (0.125)mg. At that point she will change to the lower dose size (0.125) mg. She was given a sample bottle of these tabs which should b adequate for further tapering to off I have asked her to call in a week or two for further instructions on tapering.*

3. *I have placed a call to the study coordinator to determine whether there are any specific entrance criteria and other medications to avoid so that Dianna can participate in this study.*

4. *Requisition for a referral for speech therapy. I think Dianna can benefit from this point in time especially with regard to the language functioning and further analysis of swallowing function can be done as needed.*

5. *Detailed counseling was provided. She was encouraged to call if there was any significant adverse change in her symptoms. Forty minutes for this visit, 30 of which was counseling and coordination of care.*

6. *Return to clinic in four weeks, sooner prn.*

Diagnosis: Parkinson's disease

This is the point where I began to battle the current consumer-oriented medical business. My Neurologist, Dr. XXX referred me to Dr. SSS at the University of SSS to have an evaluation for Deep Brain Stimulation. The University of SSS was the only medical facility to provide this service. I went in for two evaluations: a psychological and physical. I first underwent the psychological testing for which I passed with excellence, and the consulting resident psychologist gave me an excellent rating as a candidate for the surgery.

Deep Brain Stimulation surgery came about by a lucky accident. A neurologist in France was about to perform a pallidotomy, a surgery where certain cells are electrically overactive and these cells are cauterized to prevent the over electrical discharging, which causes the tremors. When choosing which cells to destroy, the neurologist would insert a probe that emitted a mild electric voltage. Once it was left in place too long, and to the neurologist's surprise, the subject of the surgery ceased having tremors. A company called Medtronic became aware of this accident and began focusing research to fine-tune a probe that would be connected to a battery pack, where it could be inserted via surgery into the patient's chest. The Deep Brain

Stimulator proved successful. It is currently undergoing refinements to make it more patient friendly. Is also is being tested to work for other neurophysiological illnesses.

I later had an appointment with Dr. SSS, Director of the University movement disorder clinic. After watching me walk up and down the hall once, he took my husband and me into an examining room. He did a few more neurological tests and concluded I had delayed stress syndrome due to the abuse I underwent as a child. My immediate reaction was anger. Dr. SSS tried to convince me that the brain is physically changed chemically, and it was as real an illness as Parkinson's disease. My husband then began to ask questions about delayed stress syndrome, and I sat in shocked silence as Dr. SSS detailed accounts of the effect delayed stress had on service men from the military and pictures of their MRI's showing differences in the brains. I was furious that my husband would even consider such a diagnosis as possible. I started to persist on the one point he had overlooked, that is, the one test relied on by neurologists as proof positive of a diagnosis of Parkinson's disease. "If I have delayed stress syndrome, why do I respond positively to Sinemet?" Dr. SSS modified his diagnosis to possible dopamine responsive Dystonia. Following is the summarization he wrote of our meeting to Dr. XXX:

Dear XXX,

Thank you for the consultation to see Dianna Lynn today on December 17, 2002.

She is a 49-year-old right hand woman with Parkinsonism dating back to 1989 with a right upper leg tremor. She subsequently has developed balance problems with falls. She believes her disease has progressed. She notes that she is unable to function completely without her Sinemet. She has had some freezing problems. She denies dyskinesias. She has had some dystonic posturing. Her handwriting is poor; there has been no change in facial expression.

Her review of systems reveals stress urinary incontinence and dribbling secondary to tipped uterus. There is no constipation or diarrhea. She has no dyskinesias. She has good appetite with 60-pound weight gain. She has poor handwriting. She has sleeping difficulties but no vivid dreams or hallucinations. She wears glasses. She lost hearing on the right. She had a Kidney infection and urinary tract infections in the past; there are no musculoskeletal, endocrinology, hematological, or respiratory problems. She has a benign murmur. She has had depression in the past. There are no neurological or dermatologic problems. She does have a history of significant physical abuse in the past. She had been drugged before. She had been gassed, had a garbage bag held over her head, and had blow to the head.

She is Irish background and married for 12 years. This is her second marriage. She has three children. She teaches music lessons and has 30 students presently. She obtained her BA from St. Catherine's. She had to leave school at the time of her diagnosis of Parkinsonism back then. She lives in Rosemount. She occasionally consumes alcohol, but does not smoke. She recently had a brain MRI. There are no medication allergies.

She had a tubal legation in the past. She had DeQuervain tenosnovitisdis of the right wrist and the Parkinson.

She has three sons, ages 26, 24, and 22 that are healthy. Her mother is reportedly adopted. Unclear as to the status of her father. She has a sister, who is nurse with a movement disorder, but is not clear of what the diagnosis is. She has a second sister in good health.

Her medications Sinemet 25/100, Sinemet CR 25/100, Mirapex o.5 multivitamin and COM tan 200.

Her blood pressure is 132/68, pulse 78 supine blood pressure 125/62; pulse is 119 standing and weighs 192.2 pounds.

Her carotids are regular without bruits. Her chest is clear to auscultation. Heart has regular rhythm without gallops or murmurs. Her abdominal exam is soft and contender with no masses appreciated. No peripheral edema is noted. Pulses are intact.

Her cranial nerves reveal pupils are equal, round, and reactive to light. Disks are flat Visual fields are full. Extra ocular muscles are intact. Facial sensation is normal. Sternocleidomastoid palate and tongue movements are normal. She has normal Blink. She has good facial expression. Voice volume actually is good.

She has variable tremors that are noted throughout the examination and did subside during the exams. It is unclear if this is a medication effect. There were some occasional involuntary or semi-voluntary left foot movements. She has good strength throughout with intact reflexes. There was down going toes. Sensory exam was intact X4; Heel-to-shin and finger to nose were accurate. She had a very peculiar gait. I would classify this as very atypical. As she had an astasia-abasia gait. She had impaired postural reflexes.

Impression:

Dianna Lynn is a 49 year-old, right-handed woman with a history of physical and possible sexual abuse in the past. She has a long-standing history of Parkinsonism dating back at least 13 years. It is interesting to note that she does not have prominent voice involvement. She remains to have good facial expression and blink.

The differential of her condition includes a dopamine-responsive Dystonia, conversion reaction, or a variant of idiopathic Parkinson's disease.

There are some features are somewhat unusual in her situation that makes me wonder whether or not this is idiopathic Parkinson disease.

Recommendations:
She should come in to get more testing off/on.

I would consider having her go to a North Shore in Long Island, UCLA in Los Angeles, or at Washington University of St Louis to have a Fluoro-dopa PET scan

A Neural Flouro-dopa PET scan would support a diagnosis of a conversion reaction or a dopamine responsive Dystonia. A normal PET scan would also eliminate the possibility of idiopathic Parkinson disease. An abnormal study should show selective loss in the uptake with relative sparing of the caudate. This would be supportive of Parkinson Disease. With a 13-year history, one would suspect that her PET scan would be significantly abnormal if this is idiopathic Parkinson disease or a variant of young onset Parkinson disease, which may be due to a mutation in Parkin.

Additional details about her sister's movement disorder would be very helpful in sorting out this patient's present symptoms.

ATTENTION POSSIBLE SKIN CANCER:

Additionally, the patient does have lesion on her right face that may be a squamous cell carcinoma as it seems to have some bleeding with it and a pearly border. She probably should see a dermatologist to have this evaluated.

I discussed the differential diagnosis of her condition with her and her husband. This was of course somewhat upsetting to her.

I will be happy to re-evaluate her with additional details down the road.

Please call me if there are any questions . . . .

Sincerely,
SSS
Assistant Professor of Neurology

That letter is dated December 17, 2002. My wonderful neurologist followed his recommendations to the letter. The PET scan, considered experimental, forced my neurologist to convince my HMO, HealthPartners, to pay for the test. HealthPartners is an HMO that has a reputation for putting patients' need first. Kudos to HealthPartners.

I went to New York in one day to have the Floura Dopa PET Scan. The scan did not show as normal, but the neurologist from Mount Zion stated that in his opinion, it showed that I was moderate to moderately advanced in my Parkinson's disease (please refer to exhibit). I also went in to the University Movement Disorder and had the motor testing while both off and on my drugs. I called the nurse after completing his requirements to ask whether I qualified for DBS surgery. Dr. SSS never returned my calls. My neurologist claimed to have also called and not had his calls returned. His answer was to get a third opinion. He called the Mayo clinic and set up a third referral with a former neurologist I had been able to see for two years before the HMO decided not to pay him to come to the Twin Cities anymore.

I received a letter from Dr. SSS written on June 6, 2003. I will type it exactly as it was typed:

Dear Mrs. Lynn

Thank you for coming to see us for an evaluation for Deep Brain Stimulation surgery for Parkinson's disease. The primary reason for the visit was to determine whether brain surgery is in the best interest for your Parkinson's symptoms. I will review the process that you underwent. We obtained your medical history and you underwent a neurosurgical evaluation to help us determine your diagnosis, what is your most disabling problem, any additional medical problems that would interfere with surgery, any significant medical problems or other issues that may prevent you from having a good result if you underwent surgery.

Medical history and examination findings:

You are a 49-year-old female with a 14-year history of Parkinson's symptom. You are experiencing mild, non-disabling dyskinesias, motor fluctuations, right arm and leg tremor when in the "off" state. Your symptoms began on the RIGHT SIDE.

A brain MRI was performed to look at an alternative diagnosis of Parkinson's disease, which you have been asked to repeat. The MRI was also done to evaluate for the presence of significant atherosclerosis disease (hardening of the arteries) in the brain. If present this may increase the risk of a hemorrhage (bleed)) during surgery and would therefore be a reason not to perform brain surgery.

Brain MRI result:

We have asked that you repeat the MRI as the most recent films are from 2000. These films show very prominent red nuclei, iron deposits and possibly a Chiari malformation (of which the latter is probably unrelated to your Parkinson symptoms.)

*Based on her history, you have experienced some anoxic brain injuries. Our neuroradiologist reviewed the films as well and did find evidence of anoxic brain damage; however, he did notice some the presence of iron deposits in the putamen and the sub thalamic nucleus (STN) which others have noticed. **"Again, we will need to have a repeat MRI done here at the U of SSS under our Parkinson disease protocol***

About the neuropsychological assessment, performed by Dr SSS2, this was done to evaluate for presence of significant memory difficulties, alterations in mood (for example, depression anxiety, etc.) and other factors that may make it less likely that you will benefit from surgery.

Neuropsychological evaluation:

There were mild retrieval difficulties on memory testing. Otherwise, there were no other significant performance difficulties. In fact, performance was unusually good in some areas where typical Parkinson's disease patients do fair to poor. There was also a history of "physical but not sexual abuse."

Fluorodopa (F-Dopa) Positron emission tomography (PET) scanning:

The PET scan was reviewed and it was interesting to note that the side of greater disease involvement was actually on the right side of the brain and not the left side. Your symptoms scan changes would be more severe on the left side of the brain.

Discussion

We believe that based on your history and examination, brain MRO and neuropsychological evaluation assessment that it is challenging to know what is the best management of your symptoms.

*Some unresolved issues the possibility that you have a familial movement disorder as reportedly **two sisters have movement disorders (?)**. It would be helpful for them to be evaluated and determine if their symptoms are similar. Genetic testing for you may be useful such as screening for spinocerebellar ataxias 2 and 3 (which would be unlikely if you have this), and also unlikely would be that there is a permutation in the Fragile X screen.*

Another concern is that of weight gain. You reported having gained approximately fifty pounds in one year. Most patients who undergo DBS often gain weight due to a decrease in dykinesias/movements. Our concern is that of further weight gain which could cause further medical problems and how to address that if it would occur.

If you would like to discuss this further, we would be happy to meet with you to further review and reconsider our recommendations. Another possibility is to have repeat motor testing with us administering some different medications to assess your response.

Conclusion;

Once again, we appreciate the time you spent coming to the University of SSS. Please feel free to contact us in the future for further questions. If you wish to discuss this matter face-to-face, we will have a special surgical clinic established to address this matter.

Sincerely,

Dr. SSS
Director of Movement Disorders

I was very angry and extremely upset at the number of errors in the letter and the way he came to no clear answer. He started the letter by stating correctly the reason my HMO referred me to him was for an evaluation for DBS surgery and did not fulfill his contract with my HMO by answering the question. I would not let his cavalier treatment of my illness go unanswered. I wrote him back.

August 2, 2003
RE: Dr. Sass's letter of 6/6/03 to patient Dianna Lynn

Dear Dr. SSS,

Thank you for your letter of June 6, 2003. I appreciate you taking the time to evaluate my case. You state in the opening paragraph of your letter, "The primary reason for the visit was to determine whether or not brain surgery is in the best interest for your Parkinson's symptoms." The "Conclusion" in your letter did not answer the primary reason for my referral by my HMO to your facility. In your letter, you recommended that I have an MRI at your facility. I had the recommended MRI done on July 2. As of today, Dr XXX has not received the film or the results of the MRI from your office. Your letter also listed two "unresolved issues."

The first issue discussed in our letter involved my family health history. You felt the possibility that I may have a familial disorder should be explored. On July 5, I emailed Jenny Sullivan my sister's phone number and also asked for a "Release of Information" form to send to my sister to give her neurologist to sign and return to you to allow you to review her records. I also sent a scanned copy of a death certificate of a cousin who had been diagnosed with MS who committed suicide. The death certificate indicated an autopsy was performed which will allow you to request a copy. I have not received the copy of the release of information form to send my sister and can only assume your office is assuming the responsibility for obtaining the information. I have cooperated fully with your office by providing all the information available to give you access to all information regarding my family health history.

The second issue you mentioned in your letter was regarding my weight gain. Up until a year ago I walked regularly 2 or more miles a day. Two falls resulting in a broken bone in my foot and two sprained ankles put a stop to these walks. I am also experiencing menopause. This could explain the weight gain. I had a chemically induced stress test done this month, which did not show any problems with my heart. My blood pressure and cholesterol have always registered in the low to average range.

My health care provider, HealthPartners, has been more than generous in paying for the tests for this evaluation. They paid the costs to have a Fluorodopa PET scan done for me at **your recommendation.** The PET Test has a 90% accuracy rate of correctly diagnosing persons with Parkinson's disease. The accuracy of PET scans is higher than that of neurologists who make a clinical diagnosis. My tests indicate that I have moderately advanced idiopathic Parkinson's disease. HealthPartners also paid for a MRI to be performed at your facility at a higher cost than they would have paid elsewhere. You suggest in your letter that HealthPartners pay to repeat the motor testing with different medications to assess my response. This request is unreasonable as there are hundreds of combinations of Parkinson's drugs that administered in various strengths will result in different combinations that could allow this testing to go on indefinitely.

Please correct the following error in your letter. In the paragraph under the heading "Neuropsychological evaluation," you wrote in quotes "physical but not sexual abuse." At the initial evaluation of December

7, 2002, I discussed sexual and physical abuse at some length with Dr. SSS2's intern and with you. You initially began your interview with me by suggesting that my symptoms were possibly not Parkinson's disease but were psychological because of Delayed Stress Syndrome caused by the physical and sexual abuse I underwent as a child. I became quite upset and you spoke at quite some length about how veterans came back from the war who suffered from Delayed Stress Syndrome who actually had physical changes in their brain. My husband and a student intern were in the room when this conversation took place and could verify this. Your letter should correctly read "physical and sexual abuse."

I am sure this shook the University SSS. When a doctor has disagreed or the referral does not answer the reason the patient was referred in the first place, the referring doctor would get a third opinion. This represents a loss to the HMO. I defended my HMO by following the chain of command and contacted the referring National Director for support. More patients should stand up for their health insurance carriers if they are doing an extraordinary job. One voice can make a difference if it is used to defend what is right.

The third opinion my neurologist eventually found for me confirmed my diagnosis of Young onset Parkinson's disease. He could not give an opinion on DBS, as DBS implants were not an option at his facility; he instead recommended I consider having a Parkin2 gene test completed. The name of a company that performs the gene test is Athena Diagnostics. They have a brochure that claims they can help provide answers and they were true to their word. I would strongly urge any person with a possible diagnosis of young Parkinson's disease to contact Athena Diagnostics which has a gene test for the mutations of the Parkin 2 gene. I sent in a blood sample paid for by my HMO and discovered I had two mutations, two complete deletions, in my Parkin2 gene.

Chapter 11

The Ethical Right of a Patient to a Diagnosis

In case you were wondering if I followed up on Dr. SSSS's recommendation to see a dermatologist regarding the cancerous lesion he thought he saw on my face, I did. The doctor diagnosed the lesion as cancerous and recommended surgery. He excised it in his office. A few days later, he called to let me know the lab report. Basil Carcinoma. Nevertheless, there was more to it. Apparently, the outer section of the specimen he excised also had a few cancer cells. Worried, I went back in, and he excised more skin that surrounded the lesion. This was a bit more painful. A week later, he called to tell me that this specimen was normal.

While I was going through the cancer scare, I was also sparring with one of the greatest medical names with more experience than almost anyone in treating Parkinson's disease. This person worked for one of the two or three top Parkinson Advocacy Groups in the country. He had an online column where he invited Parkinson's patients to discuss their medical issues or questions. I posted this comment because I believe every patient is entitled to any or all technology available to pin down a diagnosis. A correct diagnosis empowers the patient's doctor by giving him the information he needs to do battle with the patient's disease and predict what symptoms may come up in the future and be ready if the need arises to take action.

FDOPA SCAN

Dear Dr. So and So,

Your response to a friend who posted regarding the cost of a FDOPA scan and it's availability did not answer the question. The cost of the scan is high and its availability is low because we live in a market driven society. If doctors such as yourself do not demand the tools required to confirm the diagnosis of a disease as life altering as Parkinson's, the market will continue to be low thereby making the availability low, the cost high and medical insurance unwilling to pay the expense. The following day a second question posted was regarding FDOPA scans. Your response stated that if the diagnosis was sure that the patient had Parkinson's disease, the scan was unnecessary. A diagnosis of Parkinson's disease is never sure when the diagnosis is based on a neurologist or movement specialist opinion, even one of the best. It takes only one other neurologist to offer an opposing opinion to throw the patient into limbo. Case in point. Several neurologists, including one who treated me for two years from the Mayo clinic, have diagnosed me. All confirmed a diagnosis of Parkinson's disease. However, when I went to a local University for evaluation for Deep Brain Stimulation Therapy, the neurologist insisted I did not have PD. He insisted my symptoms were due to delayed stress syndrome because of abuse I underwent as a child. I cannot begin to tell you the pain and agony I underwent because of his diagnosis. No one should ever have to endure that type of suffering. Fortunately, I have a neurologist who was willing to submit a request for an F-DOPA Scan at Zion in New York. The results of the scan confirmed moderately advanced PD. I sent the results of the scan to the neurologist who said I did not have PD and requested him to complete my evaluation. He refused to respond. He is the only neurologist in my area certified to evaluate patients for DBS surgery.

I find your reasons for not supporting patients with PD to the most up-to-date diagnosis tool to explain

Dr. S's logic. Your expert opinion of Parkinson's disease is recognized on an international scale While you state that "diagnosis is not important, the cure is." you are causing harm to each patient in the advanced stage of the disease by not improving their quality of life. I support your position on many issues, have spoken in defense of your opinion on this site many times, and believe you have the patient's best interest at heart. On the importance of a correct diagnosis being as important as finding a cure, I am in complete disagreement.

Sincerely,
Dianna Lynn

Comment:

I appreciate your comments. I do not think pet scans are necessary: diagnosing pd better is not the issue; curing the disease is.

Another reader's response:

Diagnosing Pd better is not important? More on PET scans

Comment:

In reply to your answer: I appreciate your comments I don't think pet scans are necessary diagnosing pd better is not the issue curing the disease is"

Same Reader's Response:

Dianna's post was very powerful but to the point. What does trying to get a definitive diagnosis have to do with curing the disease? I would think even just to treat it one has to ensure that it is indeed Parkinson's and not a mimic disease much less cure the disease that I last checked was not yet possible. Even misdiagnosis rate between 10–20 percent on autopsy is excessively high. Out of the supposedly 1.5 million in the US with Parkinson's, that would put 150,000 of us as currently being misdiagnosed. Is this an acceptable statistic? Not if you are one of the150, 000. We may not yet have the technology to cure Parkinson's but we do have the technology to better diagnose it and if utilized more we could have a 100 percent diagnosis via imaging. The following reports show this as well as the many autopsy reports of Parkinson's I have read. My personal thanks to the Fox Foundation and the Parkinson's disease Foundation for supporting research in the imaging field

Comment

PD is to the PD community, and to the readers of this internet column, the major disease. But remember, PD affects 0.3 percent of the population which means 99.7 percent of the population does not have PD. PD competes with other major diseases, diabetes, heart disease, Alzheimer disease, AIDS for funds. Fluro dopa PET scan facilities are supported, in large part, by government funds, unlike MRI facilities which are not supported by public funds but by charging individual (or their insurance companies) for the test, there is not (comments from some readers notwithstanding) sufficient demand or willingness of patients or insurances to pay for pet scans (more expensive than MRIs) and, overall, less useful. Pet scan facilities especially fluro dopa facilities which require a cyclotron and support personnel are not self supporting

My turn:

F-Dopa Scan

My friend presented the case of a patient where the misdiagnosis of Parkinson's disease caused her to undergo unnecessary surgeries that caused her a strep infection in her brain. After a different doctor recommended an F-DOPA scan, which the patient did not know existed they discovered the correct diagnosis after the scan came back as normal. At this point, the Strep infection in her brain caused damage from which the patient will never recover. Had the patient had the FDOPA scan prior to the attempted DBS surgery, the patient would never have sought the surgery and would have recovered from the correct diagnosis of a disease that would have been treatable.

The harm I experienced was the doubt placed there by a doctor in whom I trusted. He is the head of Movement and Disorder Clinic at the State University in which I reside and is the only physician who does Deep brain stimulation evaluations. He is a member of your organization and recommended by you as a qualified doctor to give evaluations for DBS surgery. The doctor recommended, after giving his opinion of delayed stress syndrome, to have an FDOPA scan that my insurance paid for. It was done at the center you, yourself, have recommended as be the best and most reliable, Zion. The verdict determination is moderately advanced Parkinson's disease. Even after going to the trouble of flying to New York, a 5-hour plane ride, having the test, and flying home the same day, the doctor said he still doubted I had PD and would not approve me for the DBS surgery. I later went to a neurologist at the Mayo Clinic who cannot explain the conclusions of the University Neurologist.

Your statement in response to my last e-mail shows your eagerness to find a cure has taken priority over the basic ethical principles held by your profession. Quote from the American College of Physicians Center for Ethics and Professionalism defines the underlying principles of decision making: "These principles include beneficence, a duty to promote good and act in the best interest of the patient and the health of society, and nonmaleficence, the duty to do no harm to patients."

The misdiagnosis of Parkinson's patients is causing harm to patients.

My friend, in his last post, pointed out that the costs from treating misdiagnosed patients is borne also by society, causing harm to society in general. It is not an either/or decision, either patients are entitled accessibility to technology which improves the accuracy of their diagnosis or a cure can be found for Parkinson's disease. Both improvements of the diagnosis technique and finding a cure can be promoted. Your opinion that finding a cure for Parkinson's is more important that improving current methods of diagnosing the illness is in direct conflict with the ethical principles of your profession.

Sincerely,
Dianna Lynn

Comment:

If I had no ethical principles and I did not care about PD I would not be spending several hours each day answering questions from people with PD and providing them with relevant information for them to manage the field.

If I thought pet scans were going to be a major benefit to people with Pd I would advocate them forcefully.

When I was at the barrow I had access to a pet scan a deoxy glucose scan and used it extensively so I am not ignorant of pet scans. I found a great deal of subjectivity in reading scans and was not convinced they added greatly to what we could offer patients.

Pet scans have been available for as long or longer than MRI scans the usefulness of MRI is undisputed it's why they are so readily available if fluro dopa pet scans had the same utility they too would be universally available they are not which must tell you something

Deoxy glucose pet scans are finding a use in cancer, which is why pet scanners are more available

With regard to DBS a good neurologist and a good surgeon will recommend surgery on someone who has had a good response to levodopa not on what a pet scan shows

The question as to whether someone has or does not have dopa responsive dystonia can be answered by a trial of levodopa one does not need a pet scan

Comment 2:

I appreciate your comments I do not think pet scans are necessary. Sorry for posting twice in one day but your response to my post that brought to my attention the most severe harm your opinion, especially the one you gave to my e-mail of yesterday, to the use of FDOPA scans in diagnosing Parkinson's disease: The loss of trust between the doctor and the patient. A person on some Parkinson message boards read your response and have posted remarks about Doctor is playing God with patient's lives. Your stated position has been posted on other websites and patients are responding by expressing distrust of doctors.

My response:

Once more, the primary principle a doctor promises to uphold is to do their patient no harm. This principle must be adhered to with the same faith you approach to commune before Christ at the alter during church services. If doctors put their opinions first over the principles held to as mandatory by their profession the result is exactly what is happening in this case: loss of trust between the doctor and the patient. You must provide the best care for your patient from the diagnosis to the end state of the disease. Your energies should be focused on this goal. It is the job of the advocates to find the funds needed to find a cure. I look to God to provide the means necessary to find a cure for Parkinson's disease and if this does not happen in my lifetime I am willing to accept on faith that God alone knows the reason I must learn to accept and live with Parkinson's disease. I hate this disease and would not wish it on my worst enemy much less my children. I am unwilling to hasten the search for a cure at the expense of my fellow sufferers of this disease who have the right to demand the best care available for the diagnosis and treatment of their disease. Distrust of the patients in the Parkinson's community will only slow down the search for a cure.

Sincerely,
Dianna Lynn

Comment:

If you are distrustful of my comments then you should decease from reading them

My response:

Director:

Your response to my last post, that I should stop receiving your digest since I disagree with your ethics, was childlike. I have never questioned your medical opinion and in fact have asked you for advice in the past. When I explained what I experienced at the University Clinic shortly after its occurrence, you agreed that a FDOPA scan could be beneficial in my case. I was grateful that you encouraged me to seek further for an answer to my diagnosis rather than accept the opinion of the University neurologist that my symptoms were a result of delayed stress syndrome. I will continue to read your digest as I find a lot of helpful information both from you and from your readers. When you speak from this forum as a doctor, you are speaking as a professional who upholds in every way his Hippocratic Oath. The view you expound on regarding what technology should and should not be used when diagnosing patients is a health care management issue and you address this issue not as a Doctor but as Director of this forum which strongly influences the country on the whole of how medical management of Parkinson's Disease is treated.

I have never questioned your dedication to your patients or your profession. I do question your ethical stand on how modern technology is of use in the current management of health care. Before modern health care technology, physicians relied on their training, commonsense and experience to diagnose patients. Modern technology shows exactly what is occurring or not occurring in the patient's brain. This information provides a more reliable diagnosis from the physician who makes the decision of how to treat the patient. The doctor always has his patient's best interest in mind. He adheres to the principle to "do no harm."

The ethical problem is not the treating neurologist but the management of the health care system. The management you support refers patients to available medical technology only based on availability of pharmacological or surgical interventions. As stated in one abstract on Ethics in Medicine, "If the utility of a test is predicted on its ability to alter the behavior or action of doctors, then the test will be of little value, since there are no therapeutic options available. This line of reasoning has several consequences. First, a narrow interpretation of management leads to a disregard for other benefits that may result from innovative medical technologies.

Second, the inter-reliance between a test's utility and a physician's behavior represents a radical redirection of beneficence towards the physician and away from the patient. This results in a more rigid dichotomy between what is perceived as the needs of doctors, as opposed to the needs of patients. Finally, if the use of technology is constrained by how it does or does not change the behavior of physicians, we will have to abandon many diagnostic techniques that have not been shown to improve morbidity or mortality."

Simply put, as long as management looks only at technology in terms of how it benefits doctors and disregards how it benefits patients, it is in complete opposition of the most basic principle of medicine to allow all neurologists the opportunity to offer modern technology to patients if the neurologist believes it to be in the patients' best interest.

Your readers are mistaken to say there are only a few Parkinson suffers who disagree with your philosophy. You need only look at the professionals listed in my friend's posts on this site to understand that this issue is disturbing not only to the patients but also to many of the Neurologists in our country.

The author of the abstract from which I quoted in this message is Frederick K. Nahm, M.D., Ph.D. His education includes a residency at Harvard Medical School and Fellowship at same (Neurophysiology) and Mass. General Hospital (Neuromuscular.)

The doctors at UCLA and Zion Hospital, New York, are no less devoted to helping Parkinson's patients than you.

This issue will be resolved. Healthcare management, neurologists and concerned patients working together will resolve it. Alternatively, will it be resolved in a courtroom somewhere as another malpractice suit? Or, even worse, will the government become involved by adding further restrictions on the healthcare profession by passing more laws to protect the patient's rights?

Sincerely,
Dianna Lynn

Comment:
You have your opinion and I have mine

You did say several unkind things and you did question my integrity and dedication you can deny but you did

Pd is more than a deficiency of dopamine

If it were only a deficiency of dopamine then the current drugs would work in everyone

A pet scan can only confirm if there is deficiency of dopamine.

This can be done through a trial of Pd drugs. It does not tell you what people become demented or have difficulty with balance. Technologies such as MRI spectroscopy which measure energetices in the brain and functional MRI which tell you which centers in the brain are activated during certain movements have much more promise than fluro dopa pet scans which tell you, with a wide error, if there is a dopamine deficiency.

The government already regulates medicine and the trial lawyers have driven the costs of care up out of all proportion to any good they may have accomplished. The people who have trouble finding a movement disorder specialist know there are fewer and fewer people going into the field.

When a person persists in arguing with you it is not childish to say the two of you should go your separate ways.

After reading his perception of my e-mails, I stopped posting. As long as his perception was that I was personally attacking him rather than discussing a change in medical ethics I felt necessary, continuing to post was to no avail. I stopped posting for a year; however, there were others who kept posting mostly negative remarks.

One reader:

> *Dear Dianna,*
>
> *Enough is enough! Just in case you hadn't noticed the name of this column is "" not "Ask the director of XXX." Therefore, he is not representing anything except his opinion. Just like you have presented your view (over and over!). If you are addressing the director of XXX please use their email, mailing address, phone # etc, I thought his answers to you unbelievably restrained after your venomous attack.*
>
> *Childlike? Definitely not! As for our dear Dr., if I were him, I would simply delete your e-mails which border on harassment.*

Another reader:

Hi There,

You know folks, I have been reading and sending questions to this forum for 4 years. I was diagnosed as having PD 9 years ago. Instead of writing nasty notes to Dianna Lynn say a prayer for her. Maybe she is scared the way I am, not knowing what tomorrow will bring. Not everyone reacts to situations the same way. I just had an experience that really humbled me. I was in a chat room and was asked what illness I had. I told them PD. I asked them the same question and he told me he has colon cancer, a melanoma and a disease that he and his wife have and passed it on to their son. I felt terrible that I was complaining about having PD.

Vicki Lynn, if your reading this "Let go and let God help you, just put it in his hands. I am no religious fanatic, but I do believe in miracles, because I am one.

A group response:

> *Keep asking why, YOPA*
> *While I did not agree with Dianna Lynn and while I*
> *think this is clearly the best-informed PD forum on the*
> *'net, SHE and her friend and others were instrumental*
> *in getting an important topic addressed. Thanks to her*
> *and YOPA for not sitting still, for always asking WHY.*
> *Parkinson's is a clinical diagnosis, i.e. guess work, no*
> *matter how accomplished the treatment. It is all about*
> *asking why . . . Keep on rocking in the free world.*

Another reader's opinion:

> *I was greatly moved by the underlying factor in anger*
> *that was expressed toward you over the whole PET scan*
> *issue in today's messages.*

> *I am sorry that you had to be the focus of this anger and*
> *frustration but I commend you for the way you responded*
> *just as one would expect from a caring physician.*

> *Sometimes it seems as if doctors can work miracles and we*
> *tend to come to expect that from you and this unreasonable*
> *expectation drives the frustration and anger that some*
> *feel when your are not able to fix hat is wrong with us.*

I have written to you several times and have always appreciated your time and compassionate answers. I am new to PD (diagnosed Sept. 2003, but had symptoms for years prior to that but I am coming to grips with this new "Life companion" with the help of my dear wife and my faith in God and from caring professionals like you.

I have even come to recognize that there may be some good that comes of this disease having entered my life.

When I hear the pain and frustration and anger in Dianna Lynn's letter my heart goes out to her. I know this is a very private and personal struggle that we are all involved in but men like you help us work through it knowing we are not alone. Please don't be discouraged. Most of us do not expect a miracle from you but do respect your selfless dedication immensely.

With or without PD we can still choose to be happy in this life; we are not trapped by our quiet or not so quiet desperation. And you help many of us chose to live a full and happy life despite the presence of PD in our everyday activities.

God bless you doctor.

A reader:

>*Dear reader,*
>
>*Thank you for your note. You have more forgiveness and understanding than I and I applaud you*

My friend reappears:

>*Diagnosing PD better is not important.*
>
>*Not once have you answered any of the questions asked of you. Are you saying that the misdiagnoses rate is acceptable at 10–15%. There are tests for CANCER, AIDS, ALS, . . . etc. . . . Why is when it comes to PD experts are so sure people have it by using what I call a sobriety test. Dianna and a mutual friend and others are proven facts that the F-Dopa PETSCAN should be used in conjunction with the other diagnosing factors for PD. Or is it because DRs do not like to be proven wrong.*

Comment:

You insult me and doctors when you say we do not like to be proven wrong who but doctors did the autopsies to show that 10 to 15% of people diagnosed with idiopathic PD had something else was lewy body disease (no treatment) multiple system atrophy (no treatment)

If at this time there was a drug that STOPPED the progression of PD, then there would be a clear mandate for diagnosing the disease early and as near to 100 % as possible at present there are no such drugs.

If you go to a pd specialist he or she will tell you that they may be not be certain it's pd but return in 4 months. You cannot do that with AIDS or cancer because there are physical consequences to not instituting treatment as soon as it is diagnosed.

Comment from a recently diagnosed PD patient:

Last one, I promise:

Ashamed
Of everyone who expressed anger at Dianna Lynn for expressing her concerns.

She was a bit strong and personal but we all get that way when angry.

We all have a right to an opinion. Shame on you for attacking a fellow PWP [person with Parkinson's].

The cold fact is that up to 25% of us are misdiagnosed and some of our maladies are even curable. Trying to treat, or cure a disease without even being sure if it is the correct disease is ridiculous. How many of you have done your own research on PET or SPECT and made your own conclusions? This topic reminds me of the Pied piper, everyone listening and following without thinking for him or herself.

The final poster was a previous poster who had formerly supported the doctor. The message of patient self-education, of exploring their options and consulting with their doctor was finally getting out.

One of my all-time favorite movies is *Awakenings*, starring Robin Williams and Jeremy De Niro. Mr. Williams plays the part of the doctor, and Mr. De Niro plays the patient. The story tells of the story of paralyzed patients. Because of a rare influenza epidemic that hit the United States in the 1920s, several people were left with Parkinsonism-like symptoms to the point of paralysis. The doctor, Mr. Williams, tries to use the drug mentioned by the real-life doctor above to see if it will "awaken" the paralyzed victims from the influenza epidemic. His success led to the development of carpidopa/levodopa as we use it today. But the doctor discovered a horrible development. The drug had a short life and, if used in excess, caused uncontrollable twisting and other movements as well as had a psychological effect of causing possible anger, sadness, etc. All the patients who received the drug eventually lapsed into a similar state as they had been in before. However, the first patient woken up, Mr. De Niro, wanted his doctor to tape him and all of his symptoms as the drug was no longer working. Robin Williams is in tears at the writhing of his star patient and stopped filming. Jeremy De Niro kept urging him to continue to film, repeating one word, "Learn! Learn! Learn!" That is the role of the patient. He must share all his symptoms because the doctor only has the patients' symptoms from which to learn. The more patients the doctors examine, the more educated the doctors become. The doctors, however, must never make the mistake of sorting their patients into types. For example, I have a genetic form of PD, which is very rare. My Parkinson's progresses differently from another type such as idiopathic PD. Therefore I don't fit neatly into one of the categories. To properly treat my condition, doctors need to listen to my description of my symptoms without trying to slot me into one of the traditional categories.

Chapter 12

The Ethics of Advocacy or Can a Patient Be His Own Advocate?

Shortly after the discussion for the Ethic of a Diagnosis as a right for the patient and doctor to work together to discover a diagnosis, a reader wrote in and asked if there is any gene test for Young Onset Parkinson's patients. The reader said that he had read on another board that 50 percent of patients with Young Onset PD had a mutation in the Parkin gene. The doctor responded that such a test was too costly and only available to research patients. After almost a year, I once again posted on his web site.

The company who does testing for the Parkin gene is Athena Diagnostics. The test code is 540.

Dianna Lynn

That same day a reader jumped to the doctor's defense:

Dianna Lynn,

I believe, a journal would be an appropriate place to air your tirades, not here with Dr. I think, I can safely say to you, the rest of us reading this list, do not wish to endure your tirades anymore than Dr. wishes to do so. I would probably be correct in saying unless you have a question . . . , a KIND, pertinent comment about a post from another or news that could benefit the others in this list, do not post. There are enough stress with this illness without having to read your abusively long emails. I know, that I for one, struggle everyday to live with my diagnosis of MSA as a 32 year old woman. That, in and of itself, is more than any of us should bear. PD, MSA, other movement disorders are a cruel joke, however, I am learning to live with it and survive. Dr., I want to commend you on the fine job you do here for those of us in need of a man like you. I find, you handled this situation very well and with decorum. I apologize if I have over stepped my boundaries in your forum/ Thank you, dear sir, for this forum and your kind attention to all of us.

Sincerely,

A Reader

Comment:

Dear Reader

Thank you for your letter. Someday we all hope there will be no pd or msa and no need for this forum. I am certain Lynn also hopes for this day.

In response to a question about genetic testing for Parkinson disease, I had talked about testing for a particular gene called the Parkin 2 gene which is present in 50% of young onset people (people below age 40) with a family history, is also present in up to 20% of young onset people without a family history. I mentioned that such testing was not available commercially only in certain research labs. I was corrected, and correctly by lynn, who pointed out that Athena diagnostic labs does this test. The cost is about 500 dollars; I do not know if the test is paid for by insurance.

If you have PD (I don't know about MSA) the test tells you if there's a mutated gene (it's less clear if it tells you if you'll pass the gene on) if you don't have PD the gene does not tell you if you are at risk for pd (you may be but it can't tell you the odds)

At present the test is another piece of information and its unclear where in the puzzle for pd it fits in. The hope is researchers in the future will know more about it than now.

Comment:

Dear Dianna,
Thank you so much for the information you gave on the above gene test.

My Response:

Thank you so much for hosting such a wonderful forum which makes it possible for me to get the above info.

Genetics is a touchy ethical issue because it is so personal. Persons have a deep-seated distrust of the leak of personal information to insurance agencies, employers, or other powerful entities who could use the knowledge in a personal way. I prefer to know so that I can inform my children if they also carry the gene. I do not fall in the category spoken of above. I have two mutations of my Parkin 2 gene, deletions of exon 3 and exon 5. Now because I have two deletions, for sure each of my children will have at least one mutation. I cannot afford to pay to discover if either of my parents have a mutation, which would be the next step. If only one is from each parent, then it would be recessive. If only one of my parents has both mutations also then, it would be dominant, and all three of my children will have two mutations.

As I mentioned earlier, genetic testing is a touchy issue, even within my own family. My two elder sons are not particularly concerned. However, my younger son has told me he is a bit mad at me for making him aware of my mutations. I am involved in two gene research projects, the National Genome Project and one at the center my new neurologist works for. I am very excited to be involved in these studies as I sincerely believe our best shot at understanding the nature of diseases with Parkinson's-type symptoms is to finally have the etiology of the diseases uncovered so the researchers can find away to substitute either the correct protein or neural receptor that is missing from the patient's anatomy. Gene research is slow and exacting as every possible combination of mutations lead to different cascading events. Also it will take time and a tremendous amount of recognized genetic material to find out what triggers the mutation to go off in the wrong direction, spinning a web of errors so quickly that by the time the doctors notice something isn't right, too much damage has been done.

I knew my mother could never afford to pay for the gene test, so for the good of my children and the researchers in the genetics sciences, I called my father for the first time in over thirty years. The first call went fine. I explained to him that I would like him to discuss with his doctor the possibility of having the gene test done if his insurance would pay for it. He responded that he would be willing to pay for it if it was what I wanted. I told him no, I did not want him to pay any out-of-pocket expenses, but I knew when he retired from Fisher Body he was well insured for health. A week later, he called to tell me he had set up an appointment with his physician. He then began talking on and on about how his younger brother was an old man because he drank and did not exercise. He then began talking about how he walked every day and how young he looked for his age. Then he asked, "You'd like that, wouldn't you?" I ignored his question and asked if he would let me know when he saw his doctor and what he advised him to do. I hung up the phone, feeling dirty just for talking to him. When I was young and he would abuse me, he would always ask me if I liked it.

A few days went by, and he called again. He once more started talking about his "older" younger brother and how much younger he was. "You would like that, wouldn't you?" There was now no doubt in my mind that I had misinterpreted the last call. I asked my father had he seen his doctor and what was the doctor's advice. He countered by asking me for my address so he could send a birthday gift. I told him I barely knew him, and it was unnecessary and again asked about his doctor's advice. He told me that his doctor had told him it would not benefit him to have the test, and I thanked him for asking and hung up. I sent a few pictures of the children. I have not contacted him since.

I tried to enlighten other persons with Parkinson's disease on the young onset forums. Only a few people seemed even remotely interested in my information. The Young Parkinson's have formed an advocacy group, to which I refuse to add my voice. After refusing to agree to accept my negative views on the research of stem cell tissue on moral grounds, I was frozen out of the Parkinson's forum by the many attacks when I posted. I was accused of not understanding the issue and instructed where to read information on the subject. I had already visited and read the information posted on these sites and still could not agree with the majority. I was a problem. I was a person who was a part of a group (YOPA), could prove beyond any doubt my diagnosis even more than many of those who were members. I was not falling in line with the self-advocacy groups' principles. They seemed determined to present a united front and seemed to want my dissenting voice silenced.

I have discovered that the self-advocacy groups act much as the high school bullies I knew. They would band together and support each other. However, if anyone with different clothes, appearance, accent, or ideas showed up, they would all descend upon her/him like a flock of chickens and peck him/her to death. I argued against the use of stem cells based on my religion and was informed by one member of the forum that she was sorry I would benefit from her advocacy if stem cells led to a cure for Parkinson's disease. I assured her not to worry because I would never let that happen.

It turns out that genetics is gaining more ground due to the volunteers for genetic studies. It is much more likely she/he will benefit from my participation in gene studies.

I posted several posts regarding information I had discovered that I thought important for others with Parkinson's disease. However, if the self-advocating patients did not agree with my posts, they would begin posting polite little negative remarks until I stopped posting.

Self-advocacy groups may exist only if *all* persons who have the same disease present a unified front.

Our forefathers did not anticipate the American people to form groups with a goal in common to gang up on people who disagreed with their viewpoint. Gangs of lobbyist (advocates), some professional, have invaded our capital and are insisting on mob rule.

Parkinson's Patient Advocates sincerely believe that only they can know what it is like to live with the disease. However since no two patients with Parkinsonism present exactly the same symptoms it is difficult to form an advocacy group for Parkinson's Disease. Patients know what it is that is wrong with them and should tell the doctors about new technology that may improve the possibility of a correct diagnosis. They should take responsibility for their own health care and educate themselves about the most current information for the disease. The job of deciding how to spend research money is the job of the medical community. Their superior training, experience, and intellect make them the best voice for advising the most efficient way to spend and write grant requests for funding for patients.

Once I posted on a Parkinson's forum that I was grateful to my country for the social security disability I receive. A reader who tried to tell me it was my right to receive Social Security Disability benefits immediately scolded me. She felt she had earned hers. However, considering how long I have been receiving it, I know I never paid enough social security taxes in to pay for what I have received. The social security am being paid now comes from the taxes paid by our current workforce. I am grateful for what I receive and appreciate the generosity of today's workforce.

You do not need an advocacy or lobbyist group to have the power to make yourself heard. Just follow the rules in the current system, keep asking, moving up the chain of command until you receive the answer to your question. People are just waiting to help. Asking for help is not something to feel ashamed about. For example:

Since the Dr. SSS of the University SSS never gave the answer to what he himself stated as the primary reason for my visit, to *"determine whether or not brain surgery is in the best interest for your Parkinson's symptoms."* His conclusion in the same letter did not answer the question, *"**Conclusion:** Once again, we appreciate the time you spent coming to the University of SSS. Please feel free to contact us in the future for further questions. If you wish to discuss this matter face-to-face we will have a special surgical clinic established to address this matter."* I called on various occasions to try to set up a special surgical clinic. The unreturned phone calls indicated to me the neurologist considered his opinion as truth and would not consider me for Deep Brain Stimulation Surgery. Meanwhile my Parkinson's disease had begun taking over more of my brain, and I was experiencing severe Dystonia, so severe in my chest muscles that I could barely breathe. So I wrote to the director of the national organization to explain my dilemma and request his help:

Dear Dr.:

I have been experiencing breathing difficulties for at least a year. First, it occurred only once or twice a month when my meds wore off. The tightness in my chest would disappear completely when I took my meds.

I talked to my neurologist regarding this. He suggested increasing my meds, which I opposed as I have had PD for 16 years and have always been conservative regarding the use of drugs. After 4 or 5 months, the tightness became my primary sign that my drugs had worn off.

The pressure was quite severe, so once more I spoke to my neurologist and followed his recommendation to increase my drugs. The effect was immediate relief of the tightness in my chest. After a week, however, I began to experience constant, severe dyskinesias. I called my neurologist, as the dyskinesias were causing me a great deal of pain, and he suggested switching about four of the doses I take of regular Sinemet to Sinemet CT (Controlled Release) which I did. The dyskinesias disappeared, but once more, the pressure around my chest was unbearable so I once more resumed the higher dose he had prescribed.

The dyskinesias settled down to only happening occasionally. Now there is once more no dyskinesias and my drugs do not last long enough between doses. This past Saturday I was gasping for air, so my husband called our HMO's Consulting Nurse Line. The nurse on the phone could hear my struggle to breathe and told my husband to hang up and call 911. Fortunately, my son was at home. He also heard my attempts to breathe and came down as quickly as he could to help. My son is an EMT and currently finishing his Paramedic training. He stayed beside me and helped me to breathe slowly and evenly. The effort was exhausting me and I was about ready to give up.

My son described my attempts to breathe as "death thralls." He said there was no movement of the chest wall, only of the throat and diaphragm muscles. I was administered oxygen and a nebulizer. This would stop whatever spasmodic activity might be taking place in the bronchial tubes. The emergency room physician contacted the neurologist on call, who told him Parkinson's disease was not associated with breathing problems, and suggested sending me home with an inhaler.

On Tuesday, I was home alone when the same problem occurred. I immediately called my GP. I was talking to the nurse when once more I could only focus on trying to breathe. The nurse stayed on the phone with me to help me stay motivated to breathe. She also called 911. I was sent home with Xanex that I have been taking from my last visit to the emergency room. I saw my GP today. She said she would try to resolve the problem by Friday. Meanwhile my family is terrified to leave me home. My GP gave me permission to take a Sinemet so I do not reach the state I have been experiencing.

Since my Health Maintenance will only refer patients to Dr. SSS, who is on your recommended list of neurologists we are at a loss as to where to go to from here. The Emergency Room Physician called Dr. SSS. He instructed the Emergency Room Doctor not to increase my meds. He stated Parkinson's disease does not affect the ability to breathe.

I have read and own a copy of your book, "Shaking up Parkinson's Disease." It seems if you are referring patients who contact your foundation for a doctor to see in my state, you are referring them to a doctor who is in direct opposition to what you have written in your book.

As long as Dr. SSS continues to believe my breathing problems are not Parkinson's related (in spite of having a stress test, IKG, chest x-ray to rule out other causes) I am living in a nightmare limbo wondering if I will be able to get help the next time the ridgidity in my chest returns.

Observing the fear in my family members' eyes is more than I can take. Please call Dr. SSS and ask him to reconsider his stand on Parkinson's disease and breathing problems.

You may recall that I have written in the past regarding doctors who evaluated me for DBS and decided I do not suffer from PD. The doctor who was on call is the same doctor from the Mayo movement disorder clinic in Rochester who does not understand how Dr. SSS could arrive at his diagnosis and he assured me I do indeed have PD. I have a positive result from a SPECT Dopamine scan I had in New York at Xian Hospital, which you proclaim is the most reliable hospital to go to for fluoradopamine scans, whose result states I have moderate to moderately severe Parkinsonism. I have also tested positive for the Parkin2 gene mutation.

Dr. SSS is the only expert my HMO will approve to evaluate me for DBS. Both times I have counted on his help he has failed me.

As one Christian to another, I am begging you help him see beyond his ego, and try to help a patient who is now in a life-threatening situation and needs his help.

I will be happy to provide you copies of all documentation regarding the above. I am at a critical stage and time is getting precious to me. Please help me. If you cannot talk to Dr. SSS, perhaps you could give my GP some ideas on how to approach him.

Sincerely,
Dianna Lynn

Response:

Dear Dianna,

Shortness of breath does occur in pd but the shortness of breath described where you must go to an emergency room is not what we see in pd. There is a restriction of chest wall muscles, but when one does studies on this, the restriction is not the sort of restriction you see in conditions such as Lou gehrig's disease or the muscular dystrophies or myasthenia gravis, conditions which do result in people going to the emergency room.

Without examining you I cannot state that what I said could not apply to you. 16 years into pd is a long time. Before ascribing such severe shortness of breath to pd and increasing pd meds, I would have an ears nose and throat doctor look at you.

In some pd patients there is spasm of the vocal cords and closing of the vocal cords that shows up as shortness of breath. This should be looked into I cannot diagnose this without seeing you.

Such severe shortness of breath may also arise from a condition called pulmonary embolus in which blood clots from the veins in the legs break off and go to the lungs. PD patients, because of immobility of the legs and ridgidity of muscles of the legs, may be more prone to this.

This is something which must be looked into as it has a special treatment.

I will call the Dr and speak to him.

If a PD expert saw you in the emergency room, their first thoughts would not be that the severe shortness of breath you have is the pd; their first thoughts would be a problem with the vocal cords or a pulmonary embolism.

The doctors on our list are doctors who are usually members of the movement disorder society. When people ask my foundation about doctors, we list those who are members of the movement disorder society or heads of our centers (the center we have in your region is at Struthers). My mentioning something in my book, shortness of breath, is not the word of God in the Bible; it's a considered opinion and pd experts can and do disagree with it.

Doctor

He was as good as his word. He called and spoke to Dr. SSS to schedule an appointment to see him and, in a few weeks, his nurse called me. When I arrived for the appointment, Dr. SSS, accompanied by a psychologist, defended his first diagnosis. He denied ever receiving the letter I sent him. I asked him if he would like to look at my copy of it. He glanced at it for a few seconds. He also denied either getting any calls from my neurologist as follow-up or from me. He kept asking if he had answered all my questions every few minutes, and I could see that he was not interested in pursuing any further contact with me. He did have me speak to a geneticist who gave me a report explaining that new information had come in to make it a stronger possibility that my two mutations could be the dominant form.

When he left the room, I was in tears as I really wanted to educate him not to anger him. I did transfer over to the Struthers Parkinson's Center and began seeing a neurologist there. Struthers staff, trained to do evaluations for Deep Brain Stimulation Surgery, now offered another option for a second evaluation for DBS surgery. The hospital they were affiliated with hired a neurosurgeon qualified to do the surgery.

After that, I was able to have the DBS surgery myself. By working through the system and following the correct protocol, the current system's weaknesses became apparent and improvements in the system have been made. It only takes one person to make a change.

Chapter 13

The Self Advocacy Groups Still Don't Get the Message

Shortly afterward, I received the following mailing from the president of YOPA (Young onset Parkinson Advocates):

The American Parkinson Disease Association, Inc.

Parkinson Plaza, 135 Parkinson Avenue, Staten Island NY 10305 (718) 981-8001 (800)223-2732 Fax (718)981-4399
Educational Supplement #16

[The APDA logo was placed here.]
APDA To Ease the Burden, To Find the Cure

When Should Parkinson's Disease Patients Go To The Emergency Room?

Joseph H. Friedman, M.D.,

An emergency room (ER) physician occasionally calls to inform me that Mr. Smith is being evaluated for "freezing" or increased tremors or some other aspect of his Parkinson's disease (PD), and asked what I would advise. Usually I advise the ER doctors to tell the patient to call me the next day and get him out of the ER before anything bad happens.

A number of times I've heard the same story, "I went to the ER last week because my PD got so bad I couldn't stand it anymore! And what did they do in the emergency room? They kept me waiting six hours, did a chest x-ray, brain CT scan, cardiogram and a bunch of urine and blood tests and sent me home. And you know they didn't know anything about Parkinson's disease! They never heard of dyskinesias, of "off" periods or even some of my drugs."

It's not the ER's fault. Let's look at the role of the patient, family and perhaps PD doctors in the situation.

A trip to the ER may be useful for evaluating anything except PD. Never go to the ER because your PD is worse! You should go if you think you have an infection making the PD worse, or if you fell and are worried about a broken bone or blood clot in the brain, but if you have bad PD problems that you've been working on with your neurologist for some time, and the doctor is unavailable when your PD takes a sudden turn for the worse, I will guarantee that you will be lucky if you leave the ER with only a few hours and a few tablespoons of blood lost. ER doctors do not know much about PD. The better ones will tell you this and advise you to call your PD doctor the next day. Sometimes patients are admitted to their local hospital where their PD specialists may not be able to see them. Then someone who sees them once for 20-30 minutes alters everything that it took three years to achieve.

Now I don't mean to imply that one should never go to the ER, but I do mean that you should never go because your PD is worse without talking to your PD doctor first. Let me provide some scenarios because it is sometimes not so straightforward.

Basically, PD patients are relatively stable over weeks at a time. By this I mean optimized patients who reliably respond to the medications stay that way, perhaps developing mildly increased shuffling or tremor or dyskinesias. Patients with moderate to severe fluctuations remain fluctuating no matter how we adjust medications. If we're lucky, an adjustment will add one good hour and if we're unlucky, we may lose an hour. Some days are good, some days are bad. A person with only two good "on" hours per day may panic if there's a day without any "good" time and will experience it as a terrible, excruciatingly bad day. But in the context of the illness it really was only a little worse, 14 hours "off" increased to 16 hours "off." Of course the patient and family report that "two hours "on" went to zero," hence a complete loss of function. While this is certainly cause for grief and concern, it's not cause for alarm and all the brain CT scans and blood tests are not going to teach the ER doctors any new tricks your PD doctor doesn't already know and probably has already tried. There is no doubt that living with PD is frustrating for the patient, the caregivers and anyone else involved. No matter how many times a patient has been through an "off" to an "on" period, there is rarely a complete sense of confidence that the bad time will end. There's always a little fear that this "off" will never end and this fear, of course, makes the "off" more severe and last longer. For many patients the "on" and "off" periods are very unpredictable, making the frustration even worse. For the patient who has only small amounts of "on" time, each "on" moment is golden, so that a loss of one hour of independent mobility is a true calamity. Sometimes the frustration just boils up over the top and neither the patient nor the caregiver can take it anymore. Frequently the caregiver panics because the patient, "their responsibility", has gone downhill and there must be something the caregiver can do to fix it. Sometimes it's the patient, overcome by fear that the "on" will never happen, seeks immediate relief, as if the ER doctor can supply a remedy, like they do so easily for treating pain. Unfortunately there's no narcotic equivalent for PD. There's no magic or the patient would be on it.

When a patient whose PD has been stable suddenly deteriorates, then reasons other than the PD itself must be suspected. Pneumonia, stress, severe constipation, bladder infection, and sometimes other, more serious, non-neurologic problems may exacerbate the PD problems. The same is true for problems of memory, thinking and sleepiness. Sudden, persistent declines in concentration and memory usually indicate either an "occult" (hidden) medical problem such as an infection or thyroid dysfunction, or a medication related problem. Too often, the ER doctors diagnose "stroke" even when there's nothing to suggest this condition. They hear the words, suddenly got worse, and the one thing ER doctors know that causes sudden neurologic worsening is stroke, so the patient gets a CT scan and an unnecessary stay in the hospital. The hospital is the last place you want to be if you have problems with Parkinson's disease. (See Educational Supplement No. 5 on the hospitalization of the PD patient.) They disrupt your medication schedule, interrupt your sleep, and interfere with your exercise routines. Remember how many medication adjustments you've been through. Add one drug, subtract another, play with the schedule by a half hour, front or back load a dose of L-dopa, try physical therapy. It's unreasonable to expect an ER doctor even at the best medical centers in the country to know you or your PD better than your own doctor. No ER has a neurologist working in it. Certainly none has PD experts unless the ER doctor happens to have a family member with advanced PD. It doesn't make sense to expect a doctor who specializes in the common ER problems to know anything about PD. The ER is not a good place to get a second opinion on PD management.

Problems with PD? Call your doctor. Problems with thinking, memory, concentration, hallucinations or strange behavior? Call your PD doctor. Needless wastes of time, body fluids and money along with potential harm can be avoided with a call to the doctor who knows your PD best. Keep in mind that your doctor or a covering physician is always available but not instantly so. If you are experiencing a possible emergency then it is reasonable to expect a quick response if you let the secretary know it's urgent. However, going to an ER because the doctor didn't call back in an hour is not wise.

Copyright 1995, APDA, Inc., Reprinted Nov. 2011. Used with permission.

I am sorry, Dr. Patterson, but if I had taken your advice, "I would be standing here dead!" (quote from owner of Health Spa in movie *Dirty Dancing*.) I find your educational supplement to be demeaning to the patient, the emergency staff, and to all neurologists. I hope you are only speaking your personal opinion. The last few times I have seen my doctor at the Struthers Parkinson Center, they have had nursing staff and other medical personal sitting in on patient appointments so they can see firsthand why a patient with Parkinson's needs their medications as much as a diabetic. They are teaching hospital staff to see persons with Parkinson's disease as people, not as a disease.

Here are some excerpts from the National Parkinson's Foundation Fact Sheet. Please note what they list as their teaching goals:

FACTS ABOUT PARKINSON DISEASE:

Parkinson disease affects both men and women in almost equal numbers. It holds no social, ethnic, economic or geographic boundaries. It is estimated that four to six million people around the world suffer from the condition. In the United States, 60,000 new cases are diagnosed each year, adding to the 1.5 million Americans who currently have Parkinson disease. While the condition usually develops after age 60, approximately 15 percent of those diagnosed are under 50. Parkinson disease is estimated to cost the nation an excess of $6 billion annually, including treatment, social security payments and lost income from inability to work, according to the National Institute of Neurological Disorders and Stroke.

TRAINING PROGRAMS:

To improve the lives of persons with Parkinson disease, their caregivers and families, NPF has developed a number of signature professional training initiatives. The Allied Team Training for Parkinson program has trained dozens of professionals in several venues around the country in the proper care of Parkinson patients. The Community Partners Program seeks to identify underserved communities, forge alliances with health care providers and make available resources not otherwise known or accessible to thousands of persons needing help. Additionally, NPF sponsors a number of conferences and symposia directed at the Parkinson community of health care professionals, scientists, community leaders, patients and their families.

INFORMATION SERVICES:

Access to information on the cause, treatment and care of Parkinson disease is critical to diagnosed patients and their caregivers because of the complexity of the illness and its impact on virtually every aspect of functioning. NPF is the leading clearinghouse for information regarding all aspects of the disease and provides the latest information to persons with Parkinson disease, their families, health care professionals and the general public. NPF spends over $1,000,000 annually on its information services, which includes its website and interactive resources, the quarterly *Parkinson Report* and an extensive collection of educational manuals. All of NPF's publications are free of charge to the public and can be accessed by visiting NPF's website at www.parkinson.org.

I must apologize to the President of YOPA, but I find the American Foundation for Parkinson's disease Association, Dr. Patterson's take on hospitalization for the patient downright arrogant in opposition to the National Parkinson's Foundation's push for an avocation model.

The emergency doctors or nurses on staff do not understand the Parkinson's patient needs of his/her drugs as much as a diabetic needs their insulin and on as strict a schedule. However, Dr. Patterson, and the members of YOPA who obviously support his view, is leaving it up to the Parkinson's patient to determine or diagnose his own emergency, go to the hospital, train the staff, if they will listen, when he has a true emergency, and needs immediate medical assistance.

In June of 2005, my meds had worn off. This forced me into a barrage of dyskinesias that forced me to the floor, and I was hurting myself when I kicked the brick fireplace, the couch, bit my lip and tongue. I had absolutely no control of my body. My son is a paramedic and immediately recognized I was in shock from all the different medications I was taking. He called 911. The ambulance arrived, took me to the emergency room where the emergency room physician kept me in restrains, and heavily sedated. When the neurologist on staff arrived, she immediately had me intubated and put into a coma. I lost three days of my life in ICU. My husband said that if it were not for the quick action of the emergency staff to put me in a condition to allow the neurologist to give me life support while the Parkinson's disease drugs were flushed out of my body, I might not have made it.

I was in ICU for three days and nights. I have no memory of those days. People come up to me who visited me while I was hospitalized and I have no memory of their being at my bedside. I went through the whole procedure again about three months later. From a personal perspective, as a Parkinson's patient, I believe it is time for neurologists and advocacy groups for patients with Parkinson's disease to stop putting the decision when or if ever to go to the emergency room on the patient or their caregiver. The patient and caregiver are not medically trained to recognize an emergency. Training all hospital staff how to care for a Parkinson's patient is a more ethical way to handle this problem. There are occasions when a Parkinson's patient has symptoms that require immediate attention. Neurologists need only to consider emergencies as a possible outcome for advanced patients. The longer I have had Parkinson's disease, the less I believe it exists. I believe it is a blanket name for a number of neurophysiologic illnesses that have yet to be discovered.

I am going to relate a true story, with permission of the author, in hopes of teaching neurologists, like the one above, what happens to patients when they are denied access to well-trained hospital staff in emergency rooms. I have personally dealt with a hospital I was admitted to by contacting the director of the hospital and educating him on the importance of allowing Parkinson's patients to take their drugs on schedule. Each time I was entered into the hospital from that point on, I was provided with a twenty-four-hour round-the-clock intern to be sure my meds were administered on time.

A True Parkinson's Patient Experience

For the past week, I have been having various problems from the swelling and ulcers on my tongue to heavy-duty dyskinesias. In addition, burning pain in my fingers. It all came to a climax at about 2:00 AM Monday morning. A couple of my friends spent the night here Sunday because they were worried about me. The spastic movements got so bad that, against my protests, they took me to the ER. Almost immediately upon arrival, the ER doctor said that he had seen many cases of PD, and this was not one of them, and that I was just a "nut case." I was put into restraints, catherized, and left naked spread eagled while police, nurses, technicians and visitors strolled by and watched me writhe. He announced to me and to my friends that he was making arrangements to have me committed to a mental institution that also served as a women's prison. I begged him to call my neuro. I begged and pleaded with him to let me talk to my friends to no avail. The nurses assisting him, mocked me and told me to hold still or they would smack me. Finally, one of my friends called a neighbor, who although I don't know him, I do know his son. They called the hospital and intervened. I was sent to ICU where the nurse on duty recognized me because she had adopted a dog from me. She removed the restraints and contacted a local neuro who came and examined me immediately. He feels that there is a problem with my carbidoba/levodopa ER.

Shortly after having the restraints removed I passed out and slept for almost 12 hours. I was released yesterday.

The denial of treatment for Parkinson's patients in critical need is medical practice from the dark ages. The doctor must begin to listen to his patients and take the necessary steps to educate the medical community on some of the more serious effects of Parkinson's disease. "How can you help me if you don't believe me?"

The dialogue going on patient forums should not be mistaken for advocacy. The forums should be called a support system. The Support System on forums may be very helpful to give courage to a patient who needs to know that what symptom they are feeling is felt by others in the same position as they are. It is needed to give patients the strength to approach their neurologist with their concerns.

Up to now, patients (as groups of consumers called self-advocates) have been strongly influencing what is researched and what is not. This is America after all, and the consumer is in charge. They have directed the political system to offer grants to research only drugs or technology that will possibly affect the neurons in the substantia nigra, i.e., stem cell research, gene research, etc., and by doing so are injuring themselves and making their living quality poor. No attention has adequately been done on cascading effects, which have a huge impact on the patient's quality of life. No coordination is being done between different sciences that are also affected by loss of dopamine such as the endocrine systems, sexual abilities, psychiatric system, even the ophthalmic effects. With freedom to lobby comes responsibility. A few who belong to these patient advocacy groups were in the medical field before their Parkinson's life. They are well respected by the Parkinson's community. No two persons diagnosed with Parkinson's disease experience it exactly the same way and therefore cannot make the correct recommendations for all persons with Parkinson's disease. They are also unable to trust their cognitive skills, as Parkinson's is not just a movement disorder; it is also a psychological disease as well. Persons with Parkinson's disease must admit to themselves that their cognitive skills as well as their moods are no longer to be trusted, and they are in no position to lead the research community as *responsible* consumers and must leave determination of how and where research grants should be spent to the medical community. Persons diagnosed with Parkinson's disease, a blanket term for several movement disorders as yet undiscovered, must be responsible for individually studying all they can that pertains to their illness and educate the doctor they rely on. Because of my knowledge of my Parkin2 mutation, I knew that several completed studies had proven the DBS procedure was beneficial to those with Parkin mutations. I became a patient of the Struthers Parkinson's Center Director of Movement Disorders, Dr. Martha Nance. Dr. Nance had concerns about my having DBS surgery. She had a patient with similar symptoms and history as I who had the surgery and committed suicide. She was correctly handling my request based on her vast experience treating Parkinson's patients. I explained I understood her concern; however, I explained that every person is unique. I convinced her by reasonably stating that I was sure I would not commit suicide as it was against God's law. I would ask for help if I reached that point as I had last time I had a clinical depression. Both of us took risks in her allowing me to have surgery. My risk was assuming I knew myself better than she did and my faith in Christ was strong. She risked recommending me for the surgery against her intuition. We both were lucky and we are both happy. The surgery went well, and I am grateful for the opportunity she gave me. I did have depression. I called my psychiatrist for treatment when I found myself crying for no apparent reason several times during a week. It worked out well for me. I had researched the aftereffects of DBS surgery thoroughly. I was aware of the potential of any depression symptoms. When I started having symptoms, I immediately called my psychiatrist for treatment. I also was spiritually prepared to face whatever outcome came from having the surgery.

For me, the outcome allowed me to cut back on my drug intake, which was my goal. A negative outcome was loss of my ability to play music anymore. Playing music requires several skills that must be completed within a matter of seconds. I lost most of my fine motor movements. I practiced my clarinet when I was recovering, and after four weeks of practice, I still could not form my embouchure and play a page of music. I decided the frustration I was experiencing was no longer worth the stress caused by no progress after my continued practicing. This is when I fell into a depression. The help I received in the form of psychiatric medications helped me to be happy with what I could still do. I joined the altar guild at my church. I bought a DVD for a beginner Pilates exercise program and decided to be thankful for the wonderful years I had been able to have with my music. I must say, the Pilates DVD was a wonderful investment. I do it as soon as I get up, and the pain in the small of my back I always wake up with disappears by the end of the routine.

Chapter 14

Whose Life Is It Anyway?

There is absolutely no reason that the information obtained by testing patients' blood for Parkinson mutations should not be revealed to the patient. The information is individual, and the information will help the patient to make decisions regarding further treatment of their symptoms based on the results of DNA tests. Neurology is in its infancy, and knowing the type of mutations that patients have can help explain the patients' symptoms. The DNA mutation could tell if the cause of the symptoms is the lack or overabundance of a protein produced due to the mutation and might help to pin down a definite diagnosis. DNA is each patient's personal stamp that makes him different from every other patient.

Research companies continue to make patients sign agreements forcing them to agree to remain ignorant of the knowledge that could help them determine the best method of treating their illness. The patient is entitled to know his/her personal DNA mutations in order to make educated decisions. With the huge amount of information that can be discovered on the internet, the patient can actually research what his particular mutation means as far as his symptoms are and what research has been done to determine the most effective way to improve or maybe cure his ailment. As far as the neurologists are concerned, they do not have the time to keep up with the flood of information coming out of the consumer-driven grants and government research.

With the heavy caseload of patients and the complexity of the functioning of the brain, it is impossible for the neurologist to create an individual plan for each of his patients or diagnose with any confidence their patients' problem. If you break an arm, a doctor knows how to set it. If you suffer a heart attack, a cardiologist has a confident attitude that he can diagnose it and make recommendations to the patient to prevent another from occurring. An allergist knows how to administer several allergy tests to identify some of the standard allergies and recommend medication to help relieve the patient's discomfort. A gynecologist can help a woman prevent pregnancy. Physical therapy will help certain muscle injuries. By learning what mutation was causing my symptoms, I reclaimed my life as well as the knowledge of my individuality.

The brain is too sophisticated to allow neurologists to diagnose based on experience. Each patient has a different DNA makeup, which requires the neurologist to believe the patients' description of their symptoms or to guess by watching for patient symptoms to make a diagnosis. It could take years for all the symptoms to appear to enable a confident diagnosis. I was diagnosed with Parkinson's disease, muscular sclerosis, delayed stress syndrome, and as having no disorder, being influenced into believing I had Parkinson's disease because I had been told I had it by a neurologist. This all took place during the span of fifteen years. How can a neurologist build up trust with their patients when they do not have the tools to diagnose patients? Neurologists must not allow the researchers to continue to hoard patients' personal information that will lead to a definite diagnosis. I had stubborn faith and constant belief in my symptoms, spent hours educating myself on the internet, questioned doctors, researchers, and medical ethicists, and finally learned that there was indeed a genetic test for Young Onset Parkinson's patients that had as high as a 50 percent chance of discovering the mutation causing their symptoms that helped me to finally prove to the neurologist that I absolutely had Parkinson's disease. By obtaining the knowledge of what mutation I had, I fought for what the current studies suggested would lead to the greatest improvement of my quality of life.

At the present time, I live with Parkinson's, but it is only a part of my life. The DBS surgery permitted me to cut my drug intake to a third the amount I took before surgery. I once more feel in control of my life and of my symptoms. I am not disease free, but I do have control of my health and the decisions to improve the quality of it

I am currently able to live and deal with life's ups and downs the same as a person without Parkinson's disease. Parkinson's has been pushed to a back burner of my life for now, and I find myself focusing on living a normal life again. I am living my life on my terms and am proud of it. I pray the same for others with chronic illnesses.

AFTERWARD

It has been about 4 years since I finished this book and I wanted to bring you up to date on how I am now handling my condition. My disease has not progressed very fast. I was actually carded when at a family restaurant where I went to have pizza with my youngest son and his family. Everyone looked shocked when I was asked for ID, and I introduced my grandchildren and son. The waitress accepted my ID and we continued our meal.

I have accepted my aging with a chronic illness and no longer pursue a cure. My life quality is about as good as it gets with the help of family and friends. My husband has been overly tested during our 21+ years of marriage and has passed with flying colors. I would say a 10.0. My moods are highly unpredictable and I can go through several in a day. It has been a roller coaster ride for him but he is still with me. He and my family are proof for me of the existence of God. The love and support has helped me overcome my natural introverted personality.

I am still a pain to live with, but I am recognizing they accommodate my faults and I accommodate theirs. I accept my faults and look back at several of the fights I have fought to advocate for myself and find a very self-centered personality I regret. I took little interest in those around me in my fight to maintain a normal quality of life in not normal circumstances. I never questioned who was paying for my freedom for healthcare decisions I have demanded over the years. Freedom brings responsibility and I never chose to realize the hardship my fights had on my fellow Americans. I have been doing volunteer work which will never be enough to repay the people whom were taxed to cover my demands on the healthcare system.

The healthcare industry is overwhelmed with people like me. I want to live and have fought for survival by using more than my share of limited income. Now that I have come close to 60, I realize the burden I have become. I finished up a college degree knowing 6 months before graduation I would likely never be able to pay my government loans back adding about $15,000.00 to the national debt. I never worked long enough to earn the disability I receive monthly from Social Security. I pray for God to help our countries' leaders to make wiser decisions than I have and am living with the guilt I have placed on our countries limited income to satisfy my right to health care. I apologize to all Americans for my short sightedness in overusing my right to a quality of life of an average American who lives with a chronic illness. I cannot demand life to be fair by unceasingly demanding public money to give me back the expectations I had for my life. The illness I was unexpectedly forced to live with was what prevented me from "being all that I could be," not my fellow Americans. Life is not and cannot be fair. That is why I have my family and Faith to fall back on.

I would not change any of my past. Learning takes place in the classroom and also throughout a person's life. It comes from the struggle for survival. Because my struggle was harder than some others, my learning extracted a high price tag.

I would like to both apologize and thank my family and countrymen for the cost of my life. I could never be in a position to return the funds used over the years. I can only show my acknowledgement of my sin of selfishness by working harder to take responsibility for myself by exercising, watching what I eat, volunteering when possible, and stop focusing on my right to healthcare by externalizing my outlook on life and observing what is going on around me rather than in me.

I have never been anything but an average American but I hope those who read this self-indulgent biography will accept an apology that needed to be expressed. My kind husband has paid for the publishing of this book. No public funds have been asked for.